Identifying Neuroemergencies

Core Principles of Acute Neurology:
Recognizing Brain Injury
Providing Acute Care
Handling Difficult Situations
Communicating Prognosis
Identifying Neuroemergencies
Solving Critical Consults

Identifying Neuroemergencies

EELCO F. M. WIJDICKS, M.D., PH.D., FACP, FNCS, FANA
Professor of Neurology, Mayo Clinic College of Medicine
Chair, Division of Critical Care Neurology
Consultant, Neurosciences Intensive Care Unit
Saint Marys Hospital
Mayo Clinic, Rochester, Minnesota

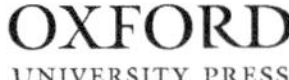

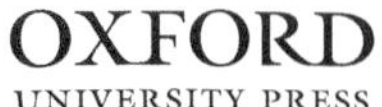

Oxford University Press is a department of the University of Oxford. It furthers the University's objective of excellence in research, scholarship, and education by publishing worldwide.

Oxford New York
Auckland Cape Town Dar es Salaam Hong Kong Karachi
Kuala Lumpur Madrid Melbourne Mexico City Nairobi
New Delhi Shanghai Taipei Toronto

With offices in
Argentina Austria Brazil Chile Czech Republic France Greece
Guatemala Hungary Italy Japan Poland Portugal Singapore
South Korea Switzerland Thailand Turkey Ukraine Vietnam

Published in the United States of America by
Oxford University Press
198 Madison Avenue, New York, NY 10016

Library of Congress Cataloging-in-Publication Data
Wijdicks, Eelco F. M., author.
Identifying neuroemergencies / Eelco F. M. Wijdicks.
p. ; cm. — (Core principles of acute neurology)
Includes bibliographical references and index.
ISBN 978-0-19-992879-8 (alk. paper)
I. Title. II. Series: Core principles of acute neurology.
[DNLM: 1. Neurologic Manifestations. 2. Central Nervous System Diseases—diagnosis.
3. Central Nervous System Diseases—therapy. 4. Emergency Medicine—methods. WL 340]
RC530
616.8′4025—dc23
2015002091

The science of medicine is a rapidly changing field. As new research and clinical experience broaden our knowledge, changes in treatment and drug therapy occur. The author and publisher of this work have checked with sources believed to be reliable in their efforts to provide information that is accurate and complete, and in accordance with the standards accepted at the time of publication. However, in light of the possibility of human error or changes in the practice of medicine, neither the author, nor the publisher, nor any other party who has been involved in the preparation or publication of this work warrants that the information contained herein is in every respect accurate or complete. Readers are encouraged to confirm the information contained herein with other reliable sources, and are strongly advised to check the product information sheet provided by the pharmaceutical company for each drug they plan to administer.

9 8 7 6 5 4 3 2
Printed in Canada

For Barbara, Coen, and Marilou

Contents

Preface

It is a singularly ubiquitous task for a neurologist in the emergency department (ED) to see a patient with acute new neurologic signs—and in this day and age, it is probably best reserved for neurohospitalists and neurointensivists. Immediately after arrival in the ED, the first course of action for the consultant is to try to identify urgency. Acute neurologic conditions have a tendency to initially present with transient or nonspecific symptoms, but that should not delude an experienced neurologist. One could say that consultation in the ED requires a heightened vigilance and a bit of healthy paranoia. There are many difficult situations, and errors can easily be made. Even more, some neurologic conditions may be nearly impossible to recognize and become apparent only after test results.

This volume is a collection of common clinical scenarios that require special attention. These constitute the majority of problems faced by the neurologist entering a loud and crowded ED. Neurologists are greatly welcomed and provide solutions to the clinical problem. Triage is another major responsibility. From the French word *trier* (to sort out), it is exactly what it implies: to find out who needs the most attention and where patients are best served. We have to continuously ask the following questions: Are we certain that triage to the ward is safe enough for the patient? What clinical neurologic conditions are difficult to recognize and why? What are the red flags? What is delayed or overlooked in the management of patients?

This volume includes the most commonly seen clinical questions with acutely ill neurologic patients in the ED, but of course not all, and other acute topics are found in the other volumes of this series. Management of acute neurologic disorders has matured through observation, practice, and more recently clinical studies. Much of what is done still is a combination of personal approach and protocol. This volume closely follows the thinking process in the ED and, I hope, provides more clarity for the practitioner and a sense of priority. In each of the presenting symptoms, I have placed figures summarizing the main differential diagnostic considerations. It remains difficult to confidently make a diagnosis in the ED in patients presenting with ambiguous signs, but in many instances, the diagnosis is clear before transport and on arrival. The one feature that all these neuroemergencies have in common is the unexpected, and this volume gives direction laying out the coordinates, so to speak. It is also useful for emergency physicians. I had their pressure and stress on my mind while putting this volume together. I very much value a close relationship between emergency physicians and neurohospitalists and neurointensivists.

At the time of this writing and at this late hour, our emergency room is filled with nearly 40 patients and among the presenting symptoms are a new seizure, headache and fever, dizziness, new leg weakness, stroke-like symptoms and a patient with hemispheric stroke and a hyperdense middle cerebral artery sign on computed tomography is on his way—the senior resident will call me soon and I will go there. I expect to see something new.

Introduction to the Series

The confrontation with an acutely ill neurologic patient is quite an unsettling situation for physicians, but all will have to master how to manage the patient at presentation, how to shepherd the unstable patient to an intensive care unit, and how to take charge. To do that aptly, the knowledge of the principles of management is needed. Books on the clinical practice of acute, emergency, and critical care neurology have appeared; but none have yet treated the fundamentals in depth.

Core Principles of Acute Neurology is a series of short volumes that handles topics not found in sufficient detail elsewhere. They focus precisely on those areas that require a good working knowledge: the consequences of acute neurologic diseases, medical care in all its aspects and relatedness with the injured brain, and difficult decisions in complex situations. Because the practice involves devastatingly injured patients, there is a separate volume on prognostication and neuropalliation. Other volumes are planned in the future.

The series has unique features. I contextualize basic science with clinical practice in a readable narrative with a light touch and without wielding the jargon of this field. The 10 chapters in each volume clearly details how things work. It is divided into a description of principles followed by its relevance to practice—keeping it to the bare essentials. There are boxes inserted into the text with quick reminders ("By the Way") and useful percentages carefully researched and vetted for accuracy ("By the Numbers"). Drawings are used to illustrate mechanisms and pathophysiology.

These books cannot cover an entire field, but brevity and economy allow focus on one topic at a time. Gone are the days of large, doorstop tomes with many words on paper but with little practical value. This series is therefore characterized by simplicity—in a good sense—with acute and critical care neurology at the core, not encyclopedic but representative. I hope it supplements clinical curricula or comprehensive textbooks.

The audience are primarily neurologists and neurointensivists, neurosurgeons, fellows, and residents. Neurointensivists have increased in numbers, and many major institutions have attendings and fellowship programs. However, these books cross disciplines and should also be useful for intensivists, anesthesiologists, emergency physicians, nursing staff, and allied healthcare professionals in intensive care units and the emergency department. In the end, the intent is to write a book that provides a sound, reassuring basis to practice well and that helps with understanding and appreciating the complexities of the care of a patient with an acute neurologic condition.

1

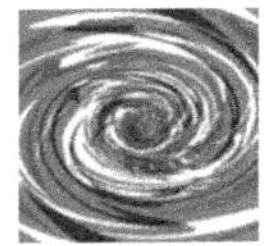

Defining Neuroemergencies

Acute neurologic disorders are everywhere in the hospital, but many patients come through the emergency department (ED). What takes precendence? The first priority is to recognize and define it as an emergency. The second priority is to successfully triage the neurologic emergency into resourceful ED and then out of it to an intensive care unit (ICU). Acute neurologic disorders are first seen either by emergency medicine services (EMS) or emergency physicians. Emergency telephone numbers (e.g., 911 in the United States) alert EMS to dispatch and to provide stabilization, followed by ground or air ambulance transport.[14,18,19,22]

Preferential triage without delay has become commonplace—patients go to the places they should go to. This concept is well established for stroke and trauma but much less established for other major emergencies (e.g., status epilepticus, central nervous system [CNS] infections), and delays or insufficient management can make a critical difference between good and bad outcomes. Even triage at the sliding door of the ED—to "critical" or not to "critical"—can make a major difference. This not-so-subtle difference determines many things such as focus on urgency, need for immediate procedures, close attention to return of laboratory results, and often a multidisciplinary approach with many healthcare workers at the bedside. Once the patient has been triaged to a critical pod of the ED, consultants will seek direction from a neurologist and will request admission and—considering the typical large volume of patients crowding the ED—rapid disposition to improve throughput.[25]

Involvement of the neurologist may come in different ways, but an urgent call to the neurologist basically already defines an acute neurologic problem. The neurologist may have previously been approached by an "outside" emergency physician facing a poorly understood condition requesting assistance. Some are in a remote area with limited capabilities and thus are requesting transfer to an ED with more resources. Resources that may be missing are often simply a neurological or neurosurgical consultation, but there may even be the inability to provide certain therapies (e.g., fresh frozen plasma, prothrombin complex concentrate [PCC], tranexamic acid). In another scenario, a patient may have been found with possible neurologic signs by the first responder, who subsequently admits the patient to the ED for immediate evaluation and support. In some of these patients, it is entirely unclear whether there is even a neurologic problem—such a determination is often left to the consulting neurologist to sort out. These are often patients seen in clinics with a presumably new neurologic problem—some may have even deteriorated right in front of the specialists' eyes (e.g., developed sudden speech impediment or possible seizure).

In the big scheme of things, neurologic problems are not a common reason for emergency evaluation (emergency physicians have to deal more frequently with presenting symptoms such as abdominal pain, chest pain, and shortness of breath).[23] Emergency physicians appreciate the additional expertise and a thorough evaluation of a neurologist—there is no doubt about that. Moreover, the privileges of the neurologist in the ED can be substantial, and often they are called on to fully manage and triage the patient.

How can the neurologist involvement work most effectively? How are urgencies recognized? What are the challenges of communication? And why are some patients different from when they were discussed over the phone? In the ED, important triage decisions should be based on fairness and how best to meet the needs of the patient (and not the needs of the physicians or institutions).[7,8,10] It is not difficult to argue that neurointensivists or dedicated neurohospitalists are in a good position to expand their role in the ED, and having such a specialized neurologist ready to see patients in the so-called golden hour may lead to improved assessment and, ultimately, to improved care and outcome. This introductory chapter addresses some of these situations in detail and provides guidance to improve initial care and triage to an ICU. It is most important to understand that many patients appear deceptively stable—until they deteriorate, that is.

Principles

A neuroemergency can be defined by the presentation of certain acute signs and also by test results, usually neuroimaging (Table 1.1). There is no doubt that there must be a major problem if there is progression, or even fluctuation, of neurologic symptoms. What is less appreciated is that improvement in symptoms may not necessarily mean the patient is improving; in fact, it may be a sign of an illness defining itself. A typical example is a patient with a basilar artery occlusion who presents with a transient hemiparesis, only to have signs of the occlusion reemerge with acute coma and new abnormalities of brainstem reflexes. Fluctuating alertness may indicate ongoing seizures. Some patients have had a nonconvulsive seizure and are in a post ictal period (they stare and are unresponsive), only to progress with a more full-blown generalized tonic–clonic seizure. Fluctuating symptoms can be a hallmark of a neuromuscular disease—myasthenia gravis is the best example.

In modern hospitals, computed tomography (CT) scanning, magnetic resonance imaging (MRI), cerebrospinal fluid (CSF) examination, and electroencephalogram (EEG) should be immediately available and could assist the neurologist greatly. CT and computed tomographic angiogram (CTA) or MRI and magnetic resonance angiogram (MRA) of the brain are mandatory to evaluate in timely fashion an

Table 1.1 **Definition of a Neurologic Emergency**

- Abnormal consciousness and coma
- Any neuromuscular respiratory failure
- Any seizure
- Any acute new headache
- Any localizing and progressing sign
- Any acute inability to stand or walk
- Any acute movement disorder
- Any CT indicating hemorrhage, mass effect, or swelling
- Any CT scan or X-ray indicating spine instability

CT = computed tomography.

emergency involving the central nervous system (CNS). MRI is very useful in the assessment of a neurologic emergency. It can be indispensable in acute spinal cord compression or any unexplained cause of coma. It is not easily available during after hours and may require special anesthesia assistance, but the neurologist can convince the (reluctant) radiologist that the test is needed and will yield important information. EEG is needed when there is clinical suspicion of seizures. In the ED, EEG is a contentious issue, as the time required to obtain one and to read it might unnecessarily delay transfer of the patient. As discussed in (Chapter 6, EEG utility in the ED is unclear and most early decisions can be made clinically. CSF examination may be underutilized (and even poorly timed when done before a CT scan); special tests may be required in patients with a CNS infection. We hope neurologists would have a say in the indication and timing of a lumbar puncture.

Of course, performance is what counts, and the major question is how this all can coalesce in practice and in the hustle and bustle of a place where emergencies come and go. The effectiveness of the neurologist in the ED is not known. Moreover, few institutions have a neurology resident in the emergency room, and even a staff neurologist may not be always physically present in the ED to assess the urgency of a case. Hospital administrators should appreciate that a neurologist with expertise in acute critical neurologic illness is best prepared to see patients who are likely going to be triaged to an ICU. Such a directive applies not only to patients admitted to specialized neurosciences ICUs (NICUs) but also to patients with acute neurologic illness who are transferred to surgical or medical ICUs or to more general ICUs. The reality is that the treatment of the "golden hour" in a neuroemergency is usually not by a neurologist, neurointensivist, or vascular neurologist. There is no easy solution—only to have a consistent 24/7 presence of a neurologist (resident with backup staff) in the ED. Teleneurology is another attractive solution. This could lead to the recognition of the need for major neurologic interventions such as a ventriculostomy placement in acute hydrocephalus, emergency MRI for a spinal cord compression, rapid treatment of status epilepticus, and treatment of mass effect with corticosteroids and osmotic diuretic agents in the appropriate most aggressive dose.[9]

Because much can go wrong before the patient even gets to the ED, it is useful here to review step by step the pathway of a patient with a neuroemergency. The first responsibility is to adequately take the patient from the out-of-hospital setting to an in-hospital setting and a face-to-face handoff with the emergency physicians. Transport decisions made at the scene by (EMS may potentially impact the outcome for patients with acute stroke and traumatic brain injury (TBI).[3] EMS know very well that neurosurgical management is only available at Level I and II trauma centers; and because of the potential need for acute intraarterial thrombolysis and endovascular clot retrieval, stroke centers are singled out for triage. However, audits have shown poor triage in TBI.[6] The American College of Surgeons Committee on Trauma (ACS-COT) and Centers for Disease Control and Prevention (CDC) have issued guidelines for field triage of injured patients. These decisions are based on level of consciousness, blood pressure, respiratory rate, anatomy of injury, mechanism of injury, and assessment within specific contexts (elderly, children, anticoagulation, pregnancy, or burns).[7] The ACS-COT accepts an overtriage rate of 50% to avoid an undertriage of ≤5%, but in reality when audited, overtriage up to 90% has been reported.[12,22] Moreover, the current situation in the United States is that a large number of patients will not be able to reach a comprehensive stroke center within 60 minutes due to the absence of emergency medical service routing policies.[15]

The first core principle of evaluation in the emergency department is to optimize patient transport. A considerable proportion of patients come from outside (far away) institutions, and travel may be problematic. Criteria for safe travel have not been clearly established for acute neurologic problems, but some guidance is provided in Table 1.2. Even a short transport by helicopter may become disastrous if a patient deteriorates during transport. Usually a combination of neurologic findings and CT abnormalities determines the mode of transport. For example, any unsecured aneurysm, recurrent

Table 1.2 **Criteria for Type of Transport in Neuroemergencies**

Air Transport	*Ground Transport*
Status epilepticus	Stable blood pressure and no IV drugs
Any major TBI	Stable airway, circulation
Any mass effect on CT	Stable stroke > 8 hours
Suspicion of CNS infection	Single seizure
Spinal cord compression	Minor or stable TBI
Hypertensive emergency	Controlled agitation
Prior anticoagulation	
Need for intubation	

TBI = traumatic brain injury; CT = computed tomography; CNS = central nervous system; IV = intravenous.

seizure, or new mass lesion with brain shift needs immediate expert care—time lost on transport should be short. Worsening from expanding hematoma or recurrent bleeding from an unsecured intracranial aneurysm may occur if anticoagulation is not reversed, blood pressure is not lowered, or antifibrinolytic drugs are not administered. Outside referring physicians should discuss appropriate airway protection in any acutely ill patient and err on the safe side. This does not apply to a patient with near-normal consciousness and orientation or a patient with a single seizure, but unfortunately many patients with questionable respiratory status are possibly inappropriately sedated, paralyzed, and intubated before transport. Neurologists should specifically ask the referring physician to go through some preparatory measures—different for each neuroemergency—before sending a patient on transport (Table 1.3).

Triage policy implementation works.[11] In a recent study in 10 stroke centers in Chicago, a triage policy resulted in an (albeit moderate) increase in tissue plasminogen activator (tPA) administration and decrease in time to onset of treatment.[18] A major recent development is the AMA/ASA stroke initiative with US hospitals qualifying as stroke centers where they provide delivery of thrombolytic agents within 60 minutes (Chapter 8). Unfortunately, only 1 in 3 of 304 target US hospitals involving over 5,000 patients reached door-to-needle time within 60 minutes.[26] Much different results were reported in northern European countries, with times approaching 20–30 minutes.[13,21] Multiple factors can cause a delay, suggesting that a broad implementation of specific time targets is needed. In the United States, citation for "poorly performing" hospitals has been considered.

The second core principle of evaluation in the emergency department is to try to get the history right. While the patient is attended to, a phone call to family

Table 1.3 **Securing Transportation to Emergency Department**

Disorder	*Considerations*
Subarachnoid hemorrhage	• 1 g tranexamic acid IV • Blood pressure control with labetalol or hydralazine (SBP < 160 mm Hg)
Cerebral hematoma	• 1 g/kg mannitol IV • Reverse anticoagulation with FFP or PCC, and vitamin K IV • Platelet transfusion with thrombocytopenia • Blood pressure control with labetalol or hydralazine (SBP < 160 mm Hg)
Traumatic brain injury	• 1 g/kg mannitol IV • Intubation and hyperventilation
Central nervous system infection	• Administer cefotaxime 2g IV, vancomycin 20 mg/kg IV, ampicillin 2 g IV, and dexamethasone 10 mg IV • Administer acyclovir 10 mg/kg IV
Brain tumor with mass effect	• Dexamethasone 10 mg IV • 1,000 mg levetiracetam IV or 20 mg/kg (fos)phenytoin IV

SBP=systolic blood pressure; IV=intravenous

members or direct communication in the ED may be essential and could provide a good sense of the time course and urgency. The information may be surprising and may result in changing course. Conditions that may seem acute may become chronic, and vice versa, after more information becomes available. Inquiries should address the use of newly introduced medication, environmental circumstances, illicit drug and alcohol use, prior neurologic illnesses, and any recent treatment for a prior major medical illness.

The third core principle of evaluation in the emergency department is to identify neurology No-No's. Neurology no-no's are summarized in Table 1.4. These are situations where an intervention or decision could worsen the patient examination or may lead to erroneous conclusions. Most situations can be avoided when there is good information about the patient's coagulation status (platelets, international normalized ratio [INR], and the use of anticoagulation), about renal function (creatinine and creatinine clearance), and about recently administered sedative drugs and neuromuscular blockers. No patient with a recent neurocatastrophe can be adequately evaluated for outcome in the ED but there are situations where the patient is moribund due to a catastrophic hemorrhage.

The fourth core principle of evaluation in the emergency department is to optimize handoffs. Insufficient communication is a problem in the ED and is related to the organizational culture and processes. As a general approach, it has been found that inadequate handoffs can lead to a diffused responsibility.[8] Some of these handoffs may be due to continuous interruptions and, in general, medical errors could be related to poor handoffs when there are communication interruptions. One study found this to occur in one of three handoffs. These interruptions lead to failure to remember what has been told. There is a tendency for physicians to overestimate the effectiveness of their handoff communication. Moreover, there is significant disagreement, when retrospectively surveyed, regarding what is the most important piece of communicated information. An important study found that ineffective handoff is a contributor to adverse clinical events and cross-coverage increased the risk of an adverse event by five times.[20] There are significant communication barriers that may relate to language and ethnic barriers and also communication style. Often there is no tool, requirement, or system to provide a standard system of communication. In addition, often there is a lack of education and a lack of training regarding how to best communicate and how to avoid interruptions and distractions in a potential chaotic environment. Most of the time, it appears that there is an inadequate amount of time for a successful handoff, with inaccurate or incomplete information provided. All of this can be remediated. A successful handoff may be taught and an example is shown in Table 1.5. This is a framework that involves the

Table 1.4 **Neurology No-No's in the Emergency Department**

- Contrast (gadolinium) in end-stage renal disease
- Lumbar puncture in coagulopathy (anticoagulants or hematologic abnormalities)
- Examination in recently sedated patient
- Prognostication or withdrawal of support in the ED (some exceptions)
- Brain death determination in recently arrived patient

Table 1.5 **The SBAR Framework**

S = Situation State what is going on with the patient and when it started
B = Background Explain the clinical background or context leading up to the situation
A = Assessment Tell what you think the problem might be
R = Recommendation State what you think needs to be done

situation, background, assessment, and recommendation (SBAR) in a simple template. Others have provided a mnemonic to synthesize information (Table 1.6). The system can also be improved by designating a specific handoff time and by using a specific place that allows sharing of detailed information. The hallway is just a bad place for communication. Some have suggested that the patient should be present during a handoff that provides instruction to the person who assumes care of the patient.

In Practice

EDs have well-thought-out policies for Level I trauma. Activation of this protocol requires tremendous available manpower, but it moves the emergency perfectly forward with increasing chances for survival of the patient (Table 1.7). In polytrauma, the neurologist is consulted once the patient is stabilized. Many EDs have a well-sorted-out stroke protocol also with the involvement of multiple personnel. Both conditions are discussed in more detail in Chapters 7 and 8.

We can expect that the physical presence of an experienced neurologist in acute neurology may result in an improved assessment, more rapid decision-making, more

Table 1.6 **Mnemonic (SIGNOUT?) in Order to Synthesize Information About the Patient**

S =	Sick or DNR? (highlight sickest patients, identify code status)
I =	Identifying data (name, age, gender, diagnosis)
G =	General hospital course
N =	New events of day
O =	Overall health status/clinical condition
U =	Upcoming possibilities with plan, rationale
T =	Tasks to complete overnight with plan, rationale
?	Any questions?

correct use of neuroimaging, and possibly better outcome.[16] Neurologists work differently in this environment and cannot move slowly and deliberately (as is often our caricatured portrayal). Here, in the ED, decisions are made on the spot without hesitation and tests are ordered with confidence expecting abnormalities, leading to necessary interventions.

ASSESSING NEUROEMERGENCIES

All physicians should consider a neurologic emergency when the patient is clearly worsening and there are changing neurologic signs. Fluctuation in hemiparesis, paraparesis, double vision, headaches, or consciousness may constitute a developing structural CNS lesion. Neurologic signs often improve before they become permanent. This simple rule applies not only to any acute vascular occlusion in cerebral or spinal cord arteries but also to a new intracranial mass. Archetypal examples are occlusion of the middle cerebral artery (MCA) stem or basilar artery that may have dramatic spontaneous resolution of major symptoms, only to get worse hours later. The mechanism here is a failing collateral system, and mild changes in blood pressure may just be enough.

Any inability to stand or walk is a neurologic emergency and may indicate a spinal cord lesion, a cerebellar hematoma, or an infarct. This simple test of having the patient stand is sometimes omitted by emergency physicians, only to have the inability discovered by a neurologist, resulting in an appropriate test to confirm clinical suspicion.

Any seizure or ongoing seizures in the ED need to be treated promptly. Benzodiazepines are the first-line therapy; intravenous (IV) lorazepam being the preferred choice because of its rapid onset of action and longer duration of antiepileptic effect. A single dose of 0.1 mg/kg of lorazepam IV immediately followed by 20 mg/kg fosphenytoin IV remains a standard approach. Midazolam can be effective in aborting

Table 1.7 **Level I Trauma Activation: Response of Staff for Initial Resuscitation of the Acutely Injured Adult Patient at Mayo Clinic**

- Trauma consultant
- Emergency physician
- Trauma critical care and general surgery junior resident or trauma physician assistant or nurse practitioner
- Radiology technician
- Phlebotomist
- Respiratory therapist
- Transfusion medicine registered nurse
- Urology technician
- Emergency medicine registered nurse

recurrent seizures only when used in high doses; and after the patient is intubated, one could administer a bolus of 0.2 mg per kilogram of body weight followed by infusion of 0.2 mg/kg/h. Transfer to the NICU is needed for prolonged and continuous EEG monitoring and to adjust medication when there is no permanent seizure control.

Acute neuromuscular respiratory weakness is not commonly seen, but often the urgency of this situation is not sufficiently appreciated. The clinical manifestations are due to failure of the pulmonary mechanics—poor lung expansion leads to reduced airflow and alveolar collapse. Atelectasis causes hypoxemia and, eventually, hypoventilation results in hypercapnia. The inadequate physiologic compensatory response increases the respiratory frequency while the tidal volumes remain small. So, when the emergency physician sees the patient for the first time, he can expect to see a patient visibly struggling to breathe, sitting up in bed, and maintaining only marginal pulse oximeter values despite increasing oxygen requirements. Myasthenic crisis is arbitrarily defined as marked worsening of limb and neck weakness with respiratory failure requiring mechanical ventilation. Myasthenic crisis may also involve a serious overdose of cholinergic drugs. (It is best remembered as SLUDGE: salivation, lacrimation, urination, defecation, gastrointestinal upset, and emesis.) Arterial blood gas measurements may or may not be informative. A relatively normal arterial blood gas may be seen in markedly fatigued patients. It may show a hypoxemic hypercapnic respiratory failure in a patient in obvious respiratory distress. However, there is more. Normally one would expect a reduced $PaCO_2$ (partial pressure of arterial CO_2) in a tachypneic patient. A normal arterial $PaCO_2$ in a tachypneic patient therefore is a sign of pending fatigue, because as a result of mechanical failure the patient cannot "blow off" CO_2. The $PaCO_2$ is "normal," only to rise when the system completely fails. (Management of neuromuscular emergencies can be found in the volume *Handling Difficult Situations*.)

INTERVENING IN NEUROEMERGENCIES

Acute neurologic illness may go through a well-known classic sequence of medical care. Neurologic examination is followed by tests (laboratory and neuroimaging) resulting in a diagnosis (often presumptive) and treatment, followed by admission for more supportive care and treatment. Examples are cerebral hemorrhage with treatment of hypertension and correction of coagulopathy in the ED before admission. Some patients are on warfarin, and this will need to be reversed immediately with vitamin K and, because of the urgency and possible surgery, with recombinant activated factor VII or PCC. This sequence can be different in other conditions. Ischemic stroke may need immediate CT scan followed by IV tPA, repeat examination, and a determination whether endovascular treatment is indicated. Similarly, treatment of a suspected CNS infection should come before all tests and diagnostic evaluations are completed to avoid treatment delay.

If there is any evidence of mass effect, shift, or edema on CT scan, intracranial pressure (ICP) is likely increased and needs to be immediately lowered. Treatment of ICP is best first managed with hyperventilation (arterial $PaCO_2$ in the 30s) and mannitol (1–2 g/kg). The use of hypertonic saline requires the placement of a central venous catheter—waiting for that to be in place could markedly delay initial treatment of

ICP. Any unsuccessful control of ICP will necessitate treatment (in patients considered eligible) with ventriculostomy followed by decompressive craniectomy, via either bifrontal craniectomy or hemicraniectomy.

Acute spinal cord compression is another neuroemergency, because immediate surgical management is needed in patients with an epidural abscess localized at a few levels, epidural hematoma, or extradural metastasis with neurologic deterioration. Its benefit lies in the preservation of at least partial mobility and, equally important, complete bladder function. Rapid decision-making regarding patients with acute spinal cord compression is paramount, because the reversal of tetraparesis or paraparesis becomes less likely with passing of time. Dexamethasone must be given to all patients with metastatic cord compression (100 mg IV push followed by 16 mg/day orally in divided doses) until definitive management has been determined.

To summarize, the sequence of events and decisions may depend on the diagnosis and several scenarios are possible (Figure 1.1). Some patients with an established diagnosis may be quickly "eyeballed" in the ED and transferred to endovascular radiology (i.e., subarachnoid hemorrhage) or NICU or operating room (lobar hematoma).

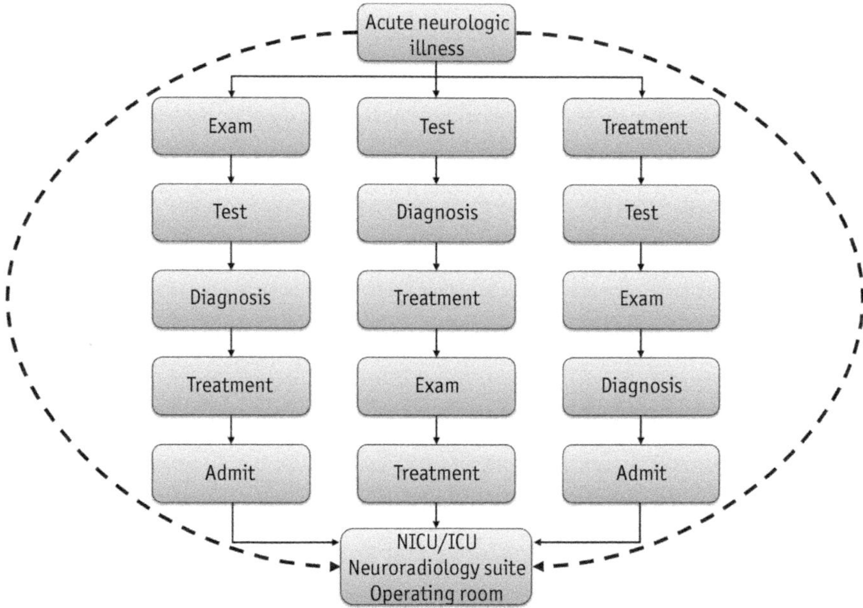

Figure 1.1 Three scenarios for emergency department triage and neurologic involvement. The left column is the traditional way of approaching a patient. In the middle column, the results of several treatments with serial tests are awaited in the ER before further triage (e.g., recurrent seizures and antiepileptic drugs). In the right column, a previously failed treatment leads to a test and eventually diagnosis and triage (e.g., acute CNS infection).

TRIAGE OF NEUROEMERGENCY

Triage to a unit or ward is based on presentation and need for a certain intervention. Triage to ICUs can be prioritized. High priority applies to all patients who could unquestionably benefit from critical care (medical or neurological). It applies to any known neurocritical illness unless a DNR order or palliative care has been decided on. For example, a patient with advanced age and a swollen dominant hemispheric infarct found at home, left alone, does not benefit from aggressive treatment either medically or surgically. Usually any neurocritical illness demands immediate treatment in the ED before triage to the ICU or NICU.[2,4,24] Many severely agitated patients may need close monitoring if treatment for agitation has been escalated. A controversial decision is whether patients who closely fulfill brain-death criteria need to be admitted for possible organ donation or should be extubated in the ED. It is a nonissue in the United States, and patients are invariably admitted. ICU "refusals" should be made only after a thorough discussion with family members—present or by phone. Most physicians would admit patients when a family asks that everything be done.[5] So unfortunately in the United States, there may be inappropriate use of ICU beds[1] and prolonged care against all odds, and this applies to all subspecialties in critical care medicine.[17] Criteria for a neurointensive care or intensive care admission include any patient with deterioration, neurologic deficit, agitation in need of repeated IV sedation, concern about respiratory support in a comatose patient, refractory seizures, additional cardiac arrhythmias or abnormal troponin, and refractory hypertension requiring IV drugs. However, a patient with an acute neurologic disease should be considered unstable; and many aspects of medical care require immediate attention. Triage suggestions are shown in Table 1.8.

Table 1.8 **Priority for Neurosciences Intensive Care or Medical Intensive Care Admission**

High (no question)	• Any established neurocritical illness • Unknown cause of coma and intubated • Status epilepticus • Acutely progressive neuromuscular disease • CT with mass effect • Neurologic disease with unstable vital signs • Neurologic disease with need for IV drugs • Neuromuscular respiratory disease • Complex endovascular procedure
Low (consider at least)	• Long-standing brain tumor with mass effect • Agitation in need of IV drugs
No (no benefit)	• DNR order and palliative care • Very sick, very old, very bad • Active refusal (patient-family)

Putting It All Together

- Neurologic emergencies often start treatment in the ED.
- There is a "golden hour" when decisions need to be made and treatment needs to be initiated.
- There are criteria for triage to the ward or ICU.
- Delay in the ED may impact outcome.
- Immediate treatment may come before definitive diagnosis.

By the Way

- Communication and handoffs may determine care in first hours.
- Triage of patients should be unbiased, transparent, and all-inclusive.
- When in doubt, just proceed with one-night stay in the ICU.
- Any patient with a cerebral mass needs an urgent neurosurgical consult.

Neuroemergency Triage by the Numbers

- ~60% of patients after aneurysmal rupture need acute ventriculostomy.
- ~50% of patients with bacterial meningitis are not treated with corticosteroids.
- ~20% of patients with Guillain–Barré syndrome (GBS) may need intubation.
- ~20% of patients with cerebral hematoma need reversal of anticoagulation.
- ~10% of spontaneous or traumatic cerebral hematomas need acute evacuation.

References

1. Angus DC, Barnato AE, Linde-Zwirble WT, et al. Use of intensive care at the end of life in the United States: an epidemiologic study. *Crit Care Med* 2004;32:638–643.
2. Azoulay E, Pochard F, Chevret S, et al. Compliance with triage to intensive care recommendations. *Crit Care Med* 2001;29:2132–2136.
3. Cameron PA, Gabbe BJ, Smith K, Mitra B. Triaging the right patient to the right place in the shortest time. *Br J Anaesth* 2014;113:226–233.
4. Escher M, Perneger TV, Heidegger CP, Chevrolet JC. Admission of incompetent patients to intensive care: doctors' responsiveness to family wishes. *Crit Care Med* 2009;37:528–532.
5. Committee SoCCME. Consensus statement on the triage of critically ill patients. *JAMA* 1994;271:1200–1203.
6. Fuller G, Lawrence T, Woodford M, Lecky F. The accuracy of alternative triage rules for identification of significant traumatic brain injury: a diagnostic cohort study. *Emerg Med J* 2014;31:914–919.
7. Gabbe BJ, Simpson PM, Sutherland AM, et al. Improved functional outcomes for major trauma patients in a regionalized, inclusive trauma system. *Ann Surg* 2012;255:1009–1015.
8. Gandhi TK. Fumbled handoffs: one dropped ball after another. *Ann Intern Med* 2005;142:352–358.

9. Hemphill JC, 3rd, White DB. Clinical nihilism in neuroemergencies. *Emerg Med Clin North Am* 2009;27:27–37, vii–viii.
10. Holliman CJ. The art of dealing with consultants. *J Emerg Med* 1993;11:633–640.
11. Kurz MW, Kurz KD, Farbu E. Acute ischemic stroke—from symptom recognition to thrombolysis. *Acta Neurol Scand Suppl* 2013;127:57–64.
12. MacKenzie EJ, Rivara FP, Jurkovich GJ, et al. A national evaluation of the effect of trauma-center care on mortality. *N Engl J Med* 2006;354:366–378.
13. Meretoja A, Strbian D, Mustanoja S, et al. Reducing in-hospital delay to 20 minutes in stroke thrombolysis. *Neurology* 2012;79:306–313.
14. Mohammad YM. Mode of arrival to the emergency department of stroke patients in the United States. *J Vasc Interv Neurol* 2008;1:83–86.
15. Moulin T, Sablot D, Vidry E, et al. Impact of emergency room neurologists on patient management and outcome. *Eur Neurol* 2003;50:207–214.
16. Mullen MT, Branas CC, Kasner SC, et al. Optimization modeling to maximize population access to comprehensive stroke centers. *Neurology* 2015;84:1–10.
17. Nelson JE, Azoulay E, Curtis JR, et al. Palliative care in the ICU. *J Palliat Med* 2012;15:168–174.
18. Prabhakaran S, O'Neill K, Stein-Spencer L, Walter J, Alberts MJ. Prehospital triage to primary stroke centers and rate of stroke thrombolysis. *JAMA Neurol* 2013;70:1126–1132.
19. Ratcliff JJ, Adeoye O, Lindsell CJ, et al. ED disposition of the Glasgow Coma Scale 13 to 15 traumatic brain injury patient: analysis of the Transforming Research and Clinical Knowledge in TBI study. *Am J Emerg Med* 2014;32:844–850.
20. Riesenberg LA, Leitzsch J, Massucci JL, et al. Residents' and attending physicians' handoffs: a systematic review of the literature. *Acad Med* 2009;84:1775–1787.
21. Sobesky J, Frackowiak M, Zaro Weber O, et al. The Cologne stroke experience: safety and outcome in 450 patients treated with intravenous thrombolysis. *Cerebrovasc Dis* 2007;24:56–65.
22. Stuke LE, Duchesne JC, Greiffenstein P, et al. Not all mechanisms are created equal: a single-center experience with the national guidelines for field triage of injured patients. *J Trauma Acute Care Surg* 2013;75:140–145.
23. Tang N, Stein J, Hsia RY, Maselli JH, Gonzales R. Trends and characteristics of US emergency department visits, 1997–2007. *JAMA* 2010;304:664–670.
24. Task Force of the American College of Critical Care Medicine, Society of Critical Care Medicine. Guidelines for intensive care unit admission, discharge, and triage. *Crit Care Med* 1999;27:633–638.
25. Traub SJ. Emergency department rapid medical assessment: overall effect and mechanistic considerations. *J Emerg Med* 2015;48:620–627.
26. Xian Y, Smith EE, Zhao X, et al. Strategies used by hospitals to improve speed of tissue-type plasminogen activator treatment in acute ischemic stroke. *Stroke* 2014;45:1387–1395.

2

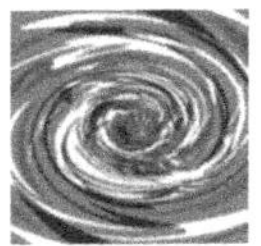

The Unresponsive Patient

Upon arrival in the ED, patients are usually marked with nondescriptive, noncategorizing, nondiagnostic labels. Such a single-phrase chief complaint—either by the patient or an accompanying family member—allows a clinical approach to the presenting symptom or sign without bias and allows open-mindedness. A typical example is the "unresponsive patient." On first impression, these patients may be comatose or not, and some may not even be unresponsive. Unresponsiveness remains one of the most common reasons for a neurologic consultation in the ED. An unresponsive patient with normal vital signs will often trigger an urgent neurologic consultation even before a CT scan is done. Thus, because the initial request for a neurologic consultation might be less specific, this chapter approaches such a presentation more broadly and more inclusively than the chapter on treatable coma in the volume *Handling Difficult Situations*. It may also further guide emergency physicians. Precise mechanisms of many of the causes of unresponsiveness are known, but a rapid neurologic assessment provides an immediate direction. Important initial questions to be asked are: Is the unresponsiveness due to coma or something else?

What are the other major neurologic disorders to consider in a suddenly unresponsive patient? How can we best initially stabilize and manage the patient, and which drugs should be used therapeutically or diagnostically? How can we quickly narrow down a differential diagnosis in acute metabolic or endocrine causes? What are the major psychiatric disorders that can produce unresponsiveness? And finally, is there something else going on that we are not aware of? These important initial questions are elaborated on in this chapter.

Principles

For lay people and first responders, the case can be made that the presence of closed eyes often points toward abnormality in level of consciousness, and when the eyes are open in an "unresponsive patient" there could be inability to communicate. However, comatose patients may have their eyes open, and alert patients may forcefully close their eyes or may not be able to open eyes due to swelling. Thus, the prominence that eye opening plays in the assessment of abnormal consciousness is not justified. Fixating objects—following objects spontaneously or to command ("tracking")—is far more useful, as we will see. The first decision to be made is whether the patient has an altered level of consciousness or not.

ASSESSMENT OF UNRESPONSIVENESS CAUSED BY COMA

The first core principle is that coma can usually only be caused by widespread brain dysfunction. Alertness is a consequence of well-functioning connecting structures—the ascending reticular activating system in the brainstem, the thalamus, and the connecting numerous fibers in the white matter—that all eventually lead to the cortex. Because of redundancy, a major shortcut is needed to cause abnormal consciousness and usually there is great damage. An example is anoxic-ischemic damage to the cortex involving the frontoparietal cortices and going into the deep vertical layers. Another mechanism is when there is diencephalic (thalamus) damage or the connection with the ascending reticular activating system is damaged. This may occur from brain shift or compression or intrinsic destruction of these crucial structures. Such a shift occurs with a large mass, but only if it appears acutely and overwhelms the system. Many large tumors may go undetected until a point of no return is reached. Clinically, this is seen as a rapid deterioration, but CT scans will then show this process has been building up for months. Sudden deterioration of a patient with a large tumor mass may be due to more swelling, acute hemorrhage into the tumor suddenly increasing the total volume, or obstruction of the ventricular system causing obstructive hydrocephalus. The impact of these progressive lesions is substantial, leaving some patients in a permanent state of unconsciousness.

Some presentations can be very much a consequence of a strategically placed lesion and not widespread injury. A lesion with the involvement of both thalami alone may lead to fluctuation of consciousness, but prolonged coma in thalamic lesions is usually seen if the lesion—whether compressive or directly destructive—extends into the mesencephalon. Akinetic mutism—a condition marked by extreme unresponsiveness with eyes fixating—is the most common clinical correlate of lesions of the anterior cingulate cortex. Involvement of the anterior cingulate gyrus is seldom seen in isolation, which is also true of lesions in the association cortex involving the precuneus and cuneus.

The second core principle is to define the depth of coma and to find a possible localization of the responsible lesion—hemispheres or brainstem or both. Such localization is only possible because we can test for brainstem reflexes. Lesions in both hemispheres generally do not produce any localizing findings until the brainstem becomes involved. Some eye findings may be seen and motor responses deteriorate to reflex movements, but not much else can help in pinpointing the degree of damage.

It is essential to first determine the response to stimuli or loud voice. Coma greatly impairs responsiveness to stimuli—deep sleep does not, and many of us can awake with some prodding (unless there is medication or alcohol ingestion). Stimuli are more and more forceful. First, the patient is gently spoken to, then yelled at, followed by "shaking," and eventually a pain stimulus (temporomandibular joint compression, nail bed compression, sternal rub) is applied. It is awful bedside manners to approach a seemingly unresponsive patient and compress a nail bed with a metal object. Several useful coma scores can be administered, but the most detailed and clinically relevant is the FOUR (Full Outline of UnResponsiveness) score (Figure 2.1).[30]

The coma scale most familiar and most used is the Glasgow Coma Scale (GCS) and is a simple scale that evaluates eye-opening, motor responses, and verbal responses (mostly testing orientation) (Table 2.1). For 40 years, it has been useful in describing unresponsiveness.[26,27] Due to little competition, it has been used ubiquitously in EDs, and surgical trauma practices.[14,19] It has some value outside the hospital, but it immediately loses its discriminatory value in intubated patients with traumatic facial swelling (both eye and verbal components become unreliable). It does not assess brainstem function.

GCS sum scores have been introduced in clinical outcome studies,[14,19] but in practice, using sum scores became rapidly problematic (e.g., GCS of 8); a low GCS score does not portend poor outcome,[13] and a high GCS score does not preclude deterioration.[10] In the United States, very few emergency physicians use the individual components in communication, and there is a strong sense among neurologists that the score is nothing more than a gross estimate rather than an actual calculation. Knowledge of the GCS is poor when actually tested in the United States and other several countries.[8,16,20,35] Most troublesome is that the motor response—often the only testable component remaining in an intubated patient with facial swelling—is often inaccurately assessed by emergency medical providers.[3]

Concerns exist with accurate use of the GCS, especially when measuring the GCS for intubated patients, who represent approximately 30%–40% of all ICU admissions. Clinicians may choose to omit the verbal component, but that will result in an incomplete score. However, an assessment of this component for a patient unable to articulate provides little value. Thus, the GCS cannot yield cogent information for intubated patients and its measurement in that group of patients is not consistent and not clearly known. (Often a "t" for tube is added resulting in V1t.) Sedation may cloud neurologic assessment and most likely would affect the GCS. The verbal component of the GCS does not address speech or language impairment. Instead, this component measures orientation and spontaneous speech, which obviously are hampered if the patient is sedated.

The FOUR score has been developed to overcome these inadequacies.[30] The number of components is four, and the maximal grade in each of the categories is also four—easy to remember and reinforced by the acronym. These four components are

1. eye responses (eye opening and eye movements),
2. motor responses (following complex commands and response to pain stimuli),
3. brainstem reflexes (pupil, corneal, and cough reflexes)
4. respiration (spontaneous respiratory rhythm or presence of respiratory drive on a mechanical ventilator).

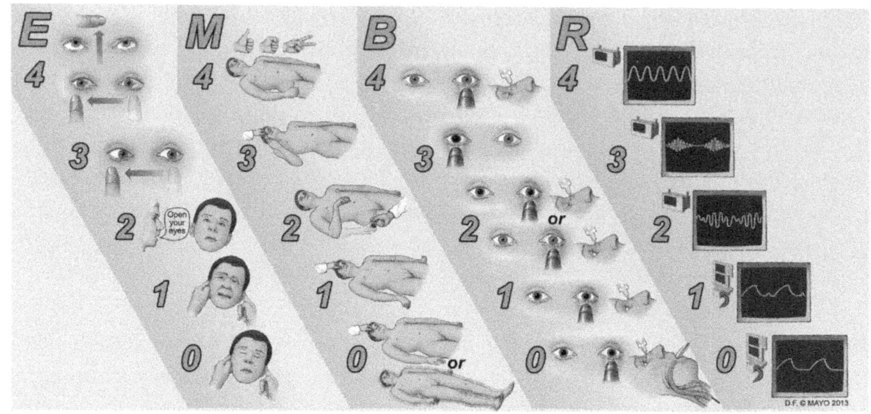

Eye response
4 = eyelids open or opened, tracking, or blinking to command
3 = eyelids open but not tracking
2 = eyelids closed but open to loud voice
1 = eyelids closed but open to pain
0 = eyelids remain closed with pain
Motor response
4 = thumbs-up, fist, or peace sign to command
3 = localizing to pain
2 = flexion response to pain
1 = extension response to pain
0 = no response to pain or generalized myoclonus status
Brainstem reflexes
4 = pupil and corneal reflexes present
3 = one pupil wide and fixed
2 = pupil or corneal reflex absent
1 = pupil and corneal reflexes absent
0 = pupil, corneal, and cough reflexes absent
Respiration
4 = not intubated, regular breathing pattern
3 = not intubated, Cheyne-Stokes breathing pattern
2 = not intubated, irregular breathing
1 = breathes above ventilatory rate
0 = breathes at ventilator rate or apnea

Figure 2.1 The FOUR score.

Table 2.1 **The Glasgow Coma Scale**

Eye Opening	*Motor Response*	*Verbal Response*
4 = Spontaneous	6 = Obeys commands	5 = Orientated
3 = To sound	5 = Localize pain	4 = Confused conversation
2 = To pain	4 = Flexion withdrawal	3 = Inappropriate words
1 = None	3 = Abnormal flexion	2 = Incomprehensible sounds
	2 = Extension	1 = None
	1 = None	

The FOUR score can be obtained in a few minutes. It does not contain a verbal component and can be measured with equal verity in intubated and nonintubated ICU patients. The three important pupil assessments in the FOUR score remain unaffected by any degree of sedation. It not only measures eye opening but also makes an assessment of voluntary horizontal and vertical eye movements. It therefore detects a locked-in syndrome in a patient with the lowest possible GCS score of 3. It detects the presence of a vegetative state, where the eyes can be spontaneously open, but do not track the examiner's finger. The motor category identifies the presence of myoclonus status (persistent widespread multisegmental arrhythmic, jerk-like movements), a poor prognostic sign in comatose patients after cardiac resuscitation. The motor component combines decorticate and withdrawal responses, because this difference is difficult to appreciate. The hand position tests (thumbs-up, fist, and peace sign) can further assess alertness, and the validity has been tested. Three brainstem reflexes test mesencephalon, pons, and medulla oblongata functions and are used in different combinations. Breathing patterns are graded. Cheyne-Stokes respiration and irregular breathing can represent bihemispheric or lower brainstem dysfunction resulting in abnormal respiratory control. In intubated patients, overbreathing of the mechanical ventilator or spontaneous breaths supported by the ventilator represents functioning respiratory centers. The FOUR score, unlike the GCS, does not include a verbal response, and thus is not only more valuable in intensive care practices that typically have a large number of intubated patients but also may be more useful in young children. Some have rightfully argued that the hand position test in the motor component already tests much of the orientation tested in the verbal score of the GCS.

In our validation studies, FOUR score assessment was good to excellent, and it predicted outcome in many patient populations[17,30,32,33] (ED, specialty and nonspecialty ICUs). Testing of each component can be easily mastered by physicians and interpreted satisfactorily by intensive care nurses. The FOUR score has also been successfully validated in the ED, which suggests that it can be used by emergency physicians at any level of training and by the nursing staff.[25] Its validity has been tested in several countries around the world and with different physicians and nursing specialties. A recent prospective study on nearly 2,000 critically ill patients found that the FOUR score is a better prognostic tool of mortality than the GCS, most likely as a result of incorporating brainstem reflexes and respiration into the FOUR score.[32] Moreover, a large multicenter prospective study of critically ill patients in the same centers previously found an excellent inter-rater agreement between paired clinicians.[11]

Using the FOUR score, the examiner is forced to describe these important, if not essential, clinical features. With all categories graded 0, the examiner is alerted to a major brain injury—assuming no confounders—and may consider a brain death examination. The FOUR score has not been tested outside the realm of acute disorders of consciousness but may also be useful in patients in a minimally conscious state and in persistent vegetative state, notwithstanding other valid coma recovery scales.

Coma scales are useful for initial assessment, but do not offer a full neurologic assessment of the comatose patient.[31] Therefore, initial neurologic assessment should include assessment of tone—rigid or flaccid or in between; assessment of breathing patterns—normal or irregular—and periodic breathing; and assessment of other brainstem reflexes, if allowed, such as oculocephalic responses. The brainstem reflexes have localizing value and the presence of anisocoria, pupillary light reflex, and reflexive motor responses indicate a structural cause of coma. Pontine lesions result in miotic pupils or are the result of organophosphate or clonidine intoxication. Any horizontal or vertical nystagmus could point to a primary brainstem lesion or cerebellar lesion compressing on the brainstem or can be seen in intoxications.

With these fundamentals, the most important questions that need to be asked by the neurologist and emergency physician[29] are as follows: Is the coma due to a destructive structural brain lesion or global acute physiological derangement of brain function; is there any structural lesion in both cerebral hemispheres or in the brainstem; or is there a lesion inside the brainstem or due to displacement of the brainstem?

Several categorical statements can be made and function as templates for diagnostic decisions[5]:

- Intrinsic brainstem lesions are recognized by skew deviation, internuclear ophthalmoplegia, small or unequal pupils, and absent oculocephalic responses.
- Brainstem displacement caused by lesions above the tentorium is recognized by a wide, fixed pupil, abnormal motor responses, but otherwise intact brainstem reflexes.
- Patients with a brainstem displacement syndrome and an abnormal CT scan often have a massive hemispheric ischemic or hemorrhagic stroke, contusional lesion, large subdural or extradural hematoma, a malignant tumor, or abscess with edema.
- Brainstem displacement from below the tentorium is recognized by small pupils, absent corneal reflexes, and absent oculocephalic responses in some patients.

- Patients with an intrinsic brainstem syndrome and a *normal* CT scan most likely have an embolus to the basilar artery.
- Patients with an intrinsic brainstem syndrome and an *abnormal* CT scan will likely show a hemorrhage in the brainstem, TBI to the brainstem, or a brainstem tumor or infectious disease.

With this information, any physician should be able to have a good sense of the nature of coma due to structural injury.

ASSESSMENT OF UNRESPONSIVENESS NOT CAUSED BY COMA

First, unresponsiveness may be related to a locked-in syndrome—it is often confused with coma but markedly different in presentation. Locked-in syndrome is uncommon and due to an acute ventral pons lesion that deafferentiates the patient for most motor function (absent horizontal eye movements, no grimacing, no swallowing, no head movements, and no limb movements). It can present as a stable deficit but can also be a transitionary state, usually when patients recover from deep unresponsive coma. It is most commonly due to acute basilar artery occlusion. Patients who are comatose have their eyes closed, whereas patients with locked-in syndrome have their eyes open, blink, and may show vertical eye movement spontaneously. Recognition of a locked-in syndrome is important because the patient might be fully aware of his surroundings but is unable to communicate other than with vertical eye movements or blinking.[31] An acute locked-in syndrome can be associated with prior use of paralytic agents and insufficient wash out but fortunately is uncommon. When the CT scan does not give an explanation (pontine hemorrhage), acute locked-in syndrome is typically due to acute ischemia of the pons from a basilar artery embolus, and an urgent cerebral angiogram by a neurointerventionalist is needed to remove the clot.

Second, some unresponsive patients are aphasic and mute. An aphasic patient is often easy to diagnose, but as a result of minimal output can be wrongly interpreted by the layperson or bystander as sudden unresponsiveness. Acute muteness may be seen in acute frontal syndrome or acute cerebellar lesion. At times, inability to speak may have a psychogenic origin or can be the result of nonconvulsive status epilepticus or dyscognitive focal seizures.[2]

Third, seizures can present with postictal agitation (and may even look like a "psychotic break") but also with unresponsiveness (and may even look like unwillingness to cooperate). Nonconvulsive status epilepticus may have unusual presentations.[24] The condition is less concerning than convulsive status epilepticus, and continuous nonconvulsive seizures likely do not cause permanent deficits.[1] Typically, the patient has fluttering eye movements and some patients have a fine nystagmus. There is often eyelid quivering and extremity twitching that can be intermittent. The patient is not blinking to threat and not following or tracking. The diagnosis is immediately made with an EEG when available in the ED. Simple caps with full montage can be placed that would allow immediate interpretation due to their online connection.[4,36,37,38] Improving technology and simplification on registration of EEG can be very helpful but would need 24/7 interpretation opportunities. It is unclear whether such use is cost-effective because nonconvulsive status epilepticus is rarely diagnosed in the ED or comes as a full surprise. Prolonged continuous EEG monitoring on the ward may have greater utility.

Fourth, another important diagnosis that should not be missed in the ED is catatonia.[9] Catatonia may have different causes and currently understood as dysregulation of the basal ganglia-thalamocortical circuit. It usually presents in a patient with a sustained posture, rigidity, mutism, and no response to any commands. On examination, waxy flexibility is found. Some patients may suddenly speak, repeat a phrase continuously (verbigeration, perseveration or stereotypes), or exhibit repetitive movements and behaviors. Some may present echopraxia (mimicking examiner's movements), echolalia (mimicking examiner's speech), paratonia (gegenhalten), or mitgehen (using slight pressure to cause the patient to move in the examiner's direction).[6,7,22,23,34] These catatonic conditions immediately respond to IV lorazepam with return to baseline within 24 hours. Most patients will have to remain on a chlordiazepoxide maintenance dose. Catatonic patients generally respond well to benzodiazepines, but other treatments may be needed to modulate glutamate and dopaminergic systems, including electroconvulsive therapy in more severe cases.[28] Acute catatonia may be mimicked by a serotonin syndrome or a neuroleptic malignant syndrome. Catatonia may also be a first manifestation of an autoimmune brain injury such as *N*-methyl-D-aspartate (NMDA) encephalopathy.[21] Most important is the significant degree of dysautonomia, which has to be aggressively treated because it can be life threatening.

Fifth, patients with Parkinson's disease or neurodegenerative disease with parkinsonian features. For example, patients with progressive supranuclear palsy may develop an akinetic crisis resulting in complete unresponsiveness. Usually, it is triggered by a viral infection, and often a surgical intervention, but it may occur without any apparent change in antidopaminergic drug administration. In fact, patients may be refractory to dopaminergic "rescue" or apomorphine IV infusion (200 mg/day). Treatment is rehydration and temperature control. Recovery is delayed.[12,18]

In Practice

"Unresponsiveness" opens up a wide array of causes, but most of them can be summarized into the 10 major causes of unresponsiveness. When the entire picture is unclear, the consulting neurologist should run through these possibilities (Figure 2.2). The first course of action is to determine whether the patient is comatose. Then one should determine whether the lesion is in one hemisphere causing mass effect (fixed dilated pupil same side of the lesion with decorticate or decerebrate motor response opposite side of the lesion), in both hemispheres (no asymmetries and often brainstem reflexes intact early on), or

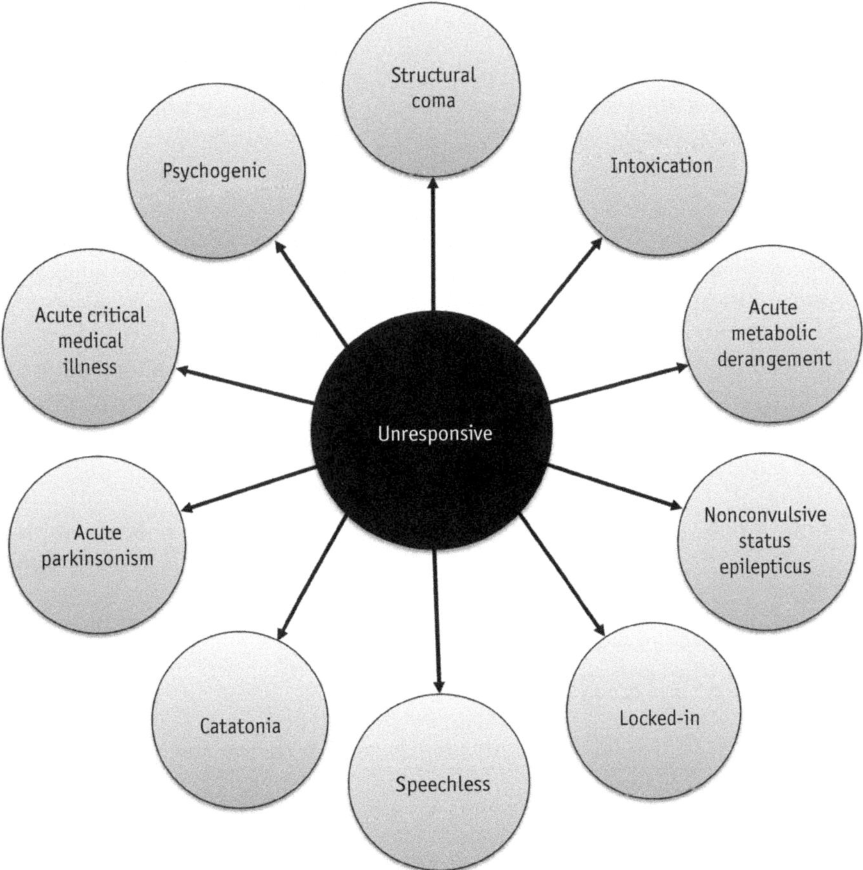

Figure 2.2 The 10 most common causes of unresponsiveness.

in the posterior fossa (pupil anisocoria and skew deviation of eye position, spontaneous vertical eye movements). This should lead to an urgent CT scan (and CTA when a basilar artery embolus is considered), and the expected lesion will be shown. If there is no vascular occlusion, mass lesion, brain edema, or acute hydrocephalus, MRI with gadolinium should be considered urgently. (MRI may demonstrate acute leukoencephalopathy, posterior reversible encephalopathy syndrome, or a brainstem infarct.) One should remember that there are many causes of structural coma that cannot be seen on CT scan. Most of these are rarities such as fat embolization syndrome, air embolization, or acute CNS infections such as meningoencephalitis.

One approach to an unresponsive patient is to immediately determine whether there is a structural brain injury that is responsible for its presentation. This can be expected in a patient with acute aphasia or muteness and a patient presenting with a locked-in syndrome. In other circumstances, unresponsiveness may not have typical neurological features, in which case an acute metabolic or endocrine derangement should be aggressively sought. Often, the type of toxin or drug a patient has ingested is known. Patients intoxicated with unknown quantities of drugs or medications present a major clinical conundrum. Helpful clinical and laboratory pointers have been developed and may assist the clinician (Table 2.2).

Drug overdoses should be treated emergently if an antidote(s) to the drug ingested is available. The six major toxidromes are cholinergic, anticholinergic, sympathicomimetic, serotonergic, narcotic, and extrapyramidal. Pupil size, blood pressure value, heart rate, and skin appearance are important determinants. Identifying the classic symptoms of a toxidrome, such as the anticholinergic toxidrome—often caused by the four "antis" of antihistamines, antipsychotics, antidepressants, and antiparkinsonians—may help expedite treatment. Unfortunately, toxidromes can be obscured by the concurrent ingestion of multiple drugs. Laboratory tests including demonstrations of quantitative levels are necessary. State of awareness may also point to certain toxins. Some toxins dampen consciousness, others cause excitation.

Often one is faced with a poorly responsive elderly patient. Some may have parkinsonian features; others may seem uncooperative and only speak when

Table 2.2 **Laboratory Abnormalities Caused by Drugs**

Hypoglycemia	Insulin, meglitinides, sulfonylureas, ackee fruit ingestion, beta blockers, ackee fruit ingestion
Hyperglycemia	Diabetic ketoacidosis, nonketotic hyperosmolar coma
Hyponatremia	Ecstasy, carbamazepine
Hypernatremia	Inadequate free water intake in setting of hypovolemia (and other states of disordered sodium homeostasis)
Hyperammonemia	Liver failure, valproic acid, urea cycle disorder
Metabolic acidosis	Methanol, ethylene glycol, paraldehyde, isoniazid, or salicylate poisoning, lactic acidosis of any cause (including cyanide and hydrogen sulfide poisoning and Wernicke's encephalopathy), ketoacidosis, uremia
Respiratory acidosis	Opioid, benzodiazepine, barbiturate
Respiratory alkalosis	Central hyperventilation, salicylates
Methemoglobinemia	Alkyl nitrites
Anion gap metabolic acidosis	Cyanide, hydrogen sulfide, toxic alcohols, salicylates, all causes of lactic acidosis
Osmolar gap	Methanol and ethylene glycol

Adapted from Edlow et al.[5]

necessary.[1] Absence of localizing neurologic findings is typical and the episode resolves. EEGs are rarely able to find nonconvulsive status epilepticus, and eventually nothing more than a severe cognitive deficit is found. Unresponsiveness may be a manifestation in advanced dementia. Unaccounted use of painkillers (opioids) should be considered.

An early CNS infection needs to be recognized because its immediate treatment could lead to immediate improvement of unresponsiveness. Most patients with an acute meningoencephalitis present with decreased consciousness and fever. In elderly and destitute alcoholics, a bacterial meningitis may not be easily recognized, and immediate coverage with multiple antibiotics is needed.[1,15]

Finally, an important cause is early sepsis in patients with an underlying dementia or neurodegenerative disease, the development of a sepsis will often lead to an acute unresponsiveness that can improve significantly with aggressive treatment. This aggressive treatment may require immediate fluid resuscitation, increase in blood pressure, and broad-spectrum antibiotics.

Psychogenic unresponsiveness in the ED remains uncommon and should only be considered if there are very specific abnormalities such as major discrepancies on examination, forced eye deviation switching with position of the approaching physician, forced eye closure, forced mouth closure, and no response to any pain stimulus while there is an absence of any brainstem involvement. Acute catatonia is a condition that needs admission to a medical ICU and psychiatry consultation.

TRIAGE

Triage of the comatose patient is to an ICU for support and treatment. Any neurosurgical lesion requires immediate transfer to the operating room. Any neurocritical illness is best transferred to an NICU (in the same hospital or elsewhere). Most episodes of unresponsiveness require further evaluation and admission to a neurology ward.

Putting It All Together

- Not all unresponsive patients are comatose.
- Most comatose patients are responsive to pain and have no localizing signs.
- Locked-in syndrome is commonly missed by physicians.
- Catatonia is commonly missed by physicians.
- Psychogenic unresponsiveness is very uncommon but easily recognized.
- Normal CT scan and unresponsiveness should lead to full laboratory testing and toxicology screening.

By the Way

- Many elderly patients have unexplained episodes of unresponsiveness.
- Alcohol use is underestimated in the elderly.
- Unauthorized self-medicating is common.
- Sudden speech arrest from seizures should be considereds in the elderly.

Unresponsiveness by the Numbers

- ~60% of acute coma is due to a structural injury to the brain.
- ~50% of acute coma in the ED is confounded by IV medication.
- ~40% of acute coma is related to cardiopulmonary resuscitation.
- ~5% of acute coma is related to prior seizures.
- ~1% of patients have a "metabolic" explanation for unresponsiveness.

References

1. Aminoff MJ. Do nonconvulsive seizures damage the brain?—No. *Arch Neurol* 1998;55:119–120.
2. Bauer G, Trinka E. Nonconvulsive status epilepticus and coma. *Epilepsia* 2010;51:177–190.
3. Bledsoe BE, Casey MJ, Feldman J et al. Glasgow Coma Scale Scoring is often inaccurate. *Prehosp Disaster Med* 2015;30:46–53.
4. Brenner RP. EEG in convulsive and nonconvulsive status epilepticus. *J Clin Neurophysiol* 2004;21:319–331.
5. Edlow JA, Rabinstein A, Traub SJ, Wijdicks EFM. Diagnosis of reversible causes of coma. *Lancet* 2014;384:2064–2076.
6. Glover SG, Escalona R, Bishop J, Saldivia A. Catatonia associated with lorazepam withdrawal. *Psychosomatics* 1997;38:148–150.
7. Greenberg K, D'Ambrosio M, Liebman KM, Veznedaroglu E. Wax on, wax off: a rare case of catatonia. *Am J Emerg Med* 2014;32:1303.e3–4.
8. Holdgate A, Ching N, Angonese L. Variability in agreement between physicians and nurses when measuring the Glasgow Coma Scale in the emergency department limits its clinical usefulness. *Emerg Med Australas* 2006;18:379–384.
9. Jaimes-Albornoz W, Serra-Mestres J. Catatonia in the emergency department. *Emerg Med J* 2012;29:863–867.
10. Joseph B, Pandit V, Aziz H, et al. Mild traumatic brain injury defined by Glasgow Coma Scale: is it really mild? *Brain Inj* 2014:1–6.
11. Kramer AA, Wijdicks EF, Snavely VL, et al. A multicenter prospective study of interobserver agreement using the Full Outline of Unresponsiveness score coma scale in the intensive care unit. *Crit Care Med* 2012;40:2671–2676.
12. Krishnan SS, Evans A, Kaye AH. Unresponsiveness due to a post surgical Parkinsonian crisis. *J Clin Neurosci* 2010;17:930–931.
13. Kushner DS. Cautionary case: low Glasgow Coma Scale scores, brainstem involvement, decompressive craniectomy, full recovery, and one more reason for advocacy/collaboration. *Am J Phys Med Rehabil* 2015;94:154–158.
14. Maas AI, Marmarou A, Murray GD, Teasdale SG, Steyerberg EW. Prognosis and clinical trial design in traumatic brain injury: the IMPACT study. *J Neurotrauma* 2007;24:232–238.

15. Michael BD, Powell G, Curtis S, et al. Improving the diagnosis of central nervous system infections in adults through introduction of a simple lumbar puncture pack. *Emerg Med J* 2013;30:402–405.
16. Namiki J, Yamazaki M, Funabiki T, Hori S. Inaccuracy and misjudged factors of Glasgow Coma Scale scores when assessed by inexperienced physicians. *Clin Neurol Neurosurg* 2011;113:393–398.
17. Okasha AS, Fayed AM, Saleh AS. The FOUR score predicts mortality, endotracheal intubation and ICU length of stay after traumatic brain injury. *Neurocrit Care* 2014;21:496–504.
18. Onofrj M, Thomas A. Acute akinesia in Parkinson disease. *Neurology* 2005;64:1162–1169.
19. Perel P, Arango M, Clayton T, et al. Predicting outcome after traumatic brain injury: practical prognostic models based on large cohort of international patients. *Bmj* 2008;336:425–429.
20. Riechers RG, 2nd, Ramage A, Brown W, et al. Physician knowledge of the Glasgow Coma Scale. *J Neurotrauma* 2005;22:1327–1334.
21. Ryan SA, Costello DJ, Cassidy EM, et al. Anti-NMDA receptor encephalitis: a cause of acute psychosis and catatonia. *J Psychiatr Pract* 2013;19:157–161.
22. Saddawi-Konefka D, Berg SM, Nejad SH, Bittner EA. Catatonia in the ICU: an important and underdiagnosed cause of altered mental status; a case series and review of the literature. *Crit Care Med* 2014;42:e234–241.
23. Shah JL, Meyer FL, Mufson MJ, Escobar JI, Goisman RM. Catatonia, conversion, culture: an acute presentation. *Harv Rev Psychiatry* 2012;20:160–169.
24. Shavit L, Grenader T, Galperin I. Nonconvulsive status epilepticus in elderly a possible diagnostic pitfall. *Eur J Intern Med* 2012;23:701–704.
25. Stead LG, Wijdicks EF, Bhagra A, et al. Validation of a new coma scale, the FOUR score, in the emergency department. *Neurocrit Care* 2009;10:50–54.
26. Teasdale G, Jennett B. Assessment of coma and impaired consciousness: a practical scale. *Lancet* 1974;2:81–84.
27. Teasdale G, Maas A, Lecky F, et al. The Glasgow Coma Scale at 40 years: standing the test of time. *Lancet Neurol* 2014;13:844–854.
28. Wachtel LE, Hermida A, Dhossche DM. Maintenance electroconvulsive therapy in autistic catatonia: a case series review. *Prog Neuropsychopharmacol Biol Psychiatry* 2010;34:581–587.
29. Wijdicks EFM. The bare essentials: coma. *Pract Neurol* 2010;10:51–60.
30. Wijdicks EFM, Bamlet WR, Maramattom BV, Manno EM, McClelland RL. Validation of a new coma scale: The FOUR score. *Ann Neurol* 2005;58:585–593.
31. Wijdicks EFM. *The Comatose Patient.* Second edition, New York: Oxford University Press; 2014.
32. Wijdicks EFM, Kramer AA, Rohs T, Jr., et al. Comparison of the FOUR Score and the Glasgow Coma Scale in predicting mortality in critically ill patients. *Crit Care Med* 2015;43:439–444.
33. Wolf CA, Wijdicks EF, Bamlet WR, McClelland RL. Further validation of the FOUR score coma scale by intensive care nurses. *Mayo Clin Proc* 2007;82:435–438.
34. Young GB. Catatonia in the ICU: something worth knowing. *Crit Care Med* 2014;42:760–761.
35. Yusuf AS, Salaudeen AG, Adewale AA, Babalola OM. Knowledge of Glasgow Coma Scale by physicians in a tertiary health institution in Nigeria. *Niger Postgrad Med J* 2013;20:34–38.
36. Zehtabchi S, Abdel Baki SG, Grant AC. Electroencephalographic findings in consecutive emergency department patients with altered mental status: a preliminary report. *Eur J Emerg Med* 2013;20:126–129.
37. Zehtabchi S, Abdel Baki SG, Malhotra S, Grant AC. Nonconvulsive seizures in patients presenting with altered mental status: an evidence-based review. *Epilepsy Behav* 2011;22:139–143.
38. Ziai W, Schlattman D, Llinas R et al. Emergent EEG in the emergency department in patients with altered mental states. *Clin Neurophysiol* 2012;123:910–917.

3

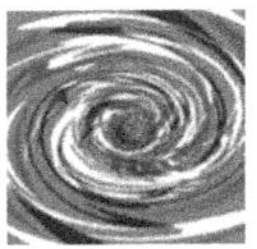

Major Warning Signs: Headache, Vertigo, Syncope

Three signs have consistently been identified by emergency physicians as the most troublesome and perhaps the most difficult to sort out in the emergency setting. Any neurologic sign can bring a patient into the ED and sound worrisome, but acute headache, sudden vertigo, and unexplained syncope often somewhat shake the confidence of emergency physicians, who would rather consult a neurologist. Emergency physicians know that acute headache may indicate subarachnoid hemorrhage (SAH), acute vertigo might indicate an acute ischemic stroke, and acute syncope might indicate seizure disorder or a life-threatening cardiac arrhythmia, though of course usually they do not. Paradoxically, it can be said that in many patients, acute headache, vertigo, or syncope have a benign cause; but it is the single patient who innocuously enters the ED and carries an acute major neurologic problem whose symptoms are wrongly interpreted or not recognized.

A known clinical problem is "anchoring," a term denoting when the emergency physician or consulting neurologist who sees the patient (often in a rush and often while multitasking in a busy ED) fixates on a certain feature too early and makes a premature assessment (Chapter 10). This happens more often in areas where less complicated disorders are often seen. A family doctor may see an SAH or cerebellar hematoma only once or twice in a decade, and some emergency physicians in remote areas may not see many more. Not being used to seeing these neuroemergencies markedly reduces diagnostic recognition, with the result that anchoring occurs ("it seems we have again a patient with severe migraine headache"). In the overwhelming proportion of patients, vertigo has a peripheral benign cause, but there is a real fear with emergency physicians that a central cause will be missed, hence a disproportionate number of consults and CT scans. Similarly, syncope is so common and so often situational or vasovagal that most neurologists are surprised that they have to see the patient urgently.

This chapter takes these important, potential warning signs and places them into clinical context. How can we best evaluate acute headache for SAH or other causes? When does acute vertigo require immediate neuroimaging

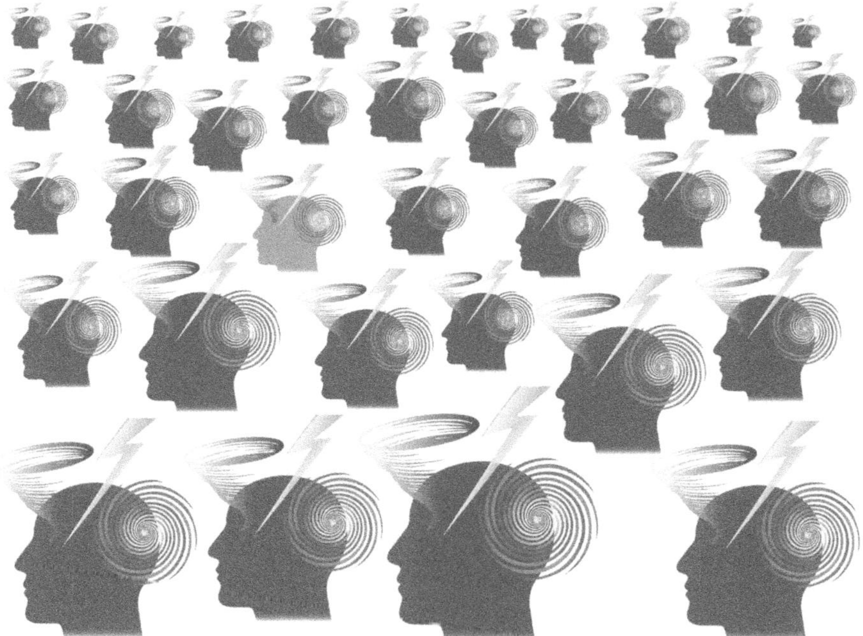

Figure 3.1 The patient with a serious illness looks uncannily identical but is still different.

for a lesion in the posterior fossa? How can we best distinguish syncope from a seizure? And how do we recognize that they may coexist? Are physicians able to identify a patient who looks much like any other patient but has a potentially life-threatening disorder ("the where is Waldo problem")? (Figure 3.1.) The literature is rife with headache, dizziness, and syncope "rules", but specificity of the tests is not great. Emergency physicians and neurologists must try to be cost-effective, more efficient, and certain rather than subjecting every patient to a battery of tests and even hospital admission.

Principles

The first core principle is that in acute headache assessment, careful analysis of the onset and character of the headache is required. So many headaches sound the same. It should be noted that in 2,000,000 patients with sufficiently severe headache in the ED, only 1 in 10 undergo neuroimaging and only 1 in 20 carry a clear neurologic diagnosis.[12]

In one neuroimaging study, the finding of an abnormality on neurologic examination increased the likelihood of a positive result threefold. Alternatively, normal findings on a neurologic examination reduced the odds of a positive finding by 30%.[19]

The common description "the worst headache of my life" is the worst description of a thunderclap headache, which is a new, split-second headache that peaks at onset. It is not known whether the history of thunderclap headache is reported accurately. The situation may be drearier when scrutinized, and a recent survey in the United Kingdom showed insufficient neurologic assessment in large numbers of patients with acute headache. Adequate history of acute headache was recorded in less than 1% of patients.[15,17] Ophthalmologic examination was not performed in 9 of 10 cases presenting in the ED when complaints are headache, visual loss, or focal signs.[5] There is no reason to think this finding does not represent most emergency rooms in the world. The only foolproof evaluation of acute, severe, totally unexpected, and previously unknown headache is a careful, detailed history of the characteristics of the headache. Examination of a patient with thunderclap headache should at least include carotid auscultation (carotid bruits may appear in carotid dissection), eye movements (for cranial nerve deficits), neck movement (for neck stiffness), and ophthalmoscopy (for hypertensive retinopathy in posterior reversible encephalopathy syndrome, retinal hemorrhage, or Terson's syndrome).

Most patients will confirm the headache is acute; but when pressed, and the acuteness is demonstrated by a loud handclap, many patients describe the headache as building up gradually in a matter of minutes. A thunderclap headache is typically completely different from prior headaches. It may be labeled by the patient as the worst headache, but most "worst headaches" are migraine relapses rather than a ruptured aneurysm. Headache associated with SAH is commonly found, although some patients with SAH do not recall headaches because they experienced loss of consciousness.

There are additional signs and symptoms that would point toward an acute SAH. The so-called Ottawa SAH rule appears to have high sensitivity. This rule includes the following: It is first assumed that there is no prior neurologic disorder that could have caused the headache. Second, there are high-risk variables that include age more than 40 years, neck pain or stiffness, witnessed loss of consciousness, onset during exertion or sexual activity, instantly peaking pain, and limited neck flexion on examination. The rule is 100% sensitive and 15% specific in detecting SAH in patients with acute headache, a normal examination and maximal intensity of headache to 1 hour.[16,18] Validation in another set of patients confirmed 100% sensitivity but much lower specificity at nearly 8%.[2] The rule may not be applicable to most patients seen in the ED.

No emergency physician or neurologist would defer a CT scan in any new headache even if the pretest probability was low, but the real pending question is whether these factors could determine the need for a lumbar puncture when CT scan is normal. Only about 4 of 3,000 patients who received a lumbar puncture for headache are diagnosed with SAH after a normal CT scan.[8,10]

Generally, acute thunderclap headache still requires a lumbar puncture. Essentially, the risk of missing an SAH with a normal CT scan performed 6 hours after onset is less than 1% when CT is evaluated by a neuroradiologist. Moreover, lumbar puncture can be easily traumatic. (This occurs in obese patients who have poorly identified spine processes that make palpability problematic and, therefore, present a higher likelihood of traumatic taps. When spine processes are difficult to palpate, fluoroscopy guidance is important to reduce traumatic dural punctures.[11]) In any situation, a CT scan should be performed first, carefully scrutinized for areas where SAH might be present and reviewed by others if doubt exists, and then followed by a lumbar puncture. Xanthochromia is typically noted after visual inspection. Many EU countries and the United Kingdom use spectrophotometry to further detect the presence of bilirubin or oxyhemoglobin; however, the reliability and specificity may be even less than visual inspection.[8] A CTA can be considered in these patients, but it rarely goes beyond 95% sensitivity and is often lower. Some of these patients may have small dissecting cerebral aneurysms of perforators and they are easy to miss on CTA. Cerebral angiogram remains the gold standard for finding a possible ruptured cerebral aneurysm.

The second core principle is that acute headaches can occur with other neurologic disorders. Acute severe headache may indicate a cerebellar hematoma, possibly an expanding dissecting not yet ruptured intracranial aneurysm, carotid or vertebral artery dissection, and pituitary apoplexy. Acute headache may be due to nonneurologic causes. Neurologists should be aware that acute, severe headaches might be due to acute angle glaucoma, temporal arteritis, acute sinusitis, or herpes zoster ophthalmicus, and in rare cases associated with hypertensive crisis. None of the time profiles are specific, nor are there characteristic features that could distinguish between any of these headache syndromes. The most important considerations with acute headaches to consider in the ED are shown in Figure 3.2-less common but equally important causes to consider are shown in Table 3.1.

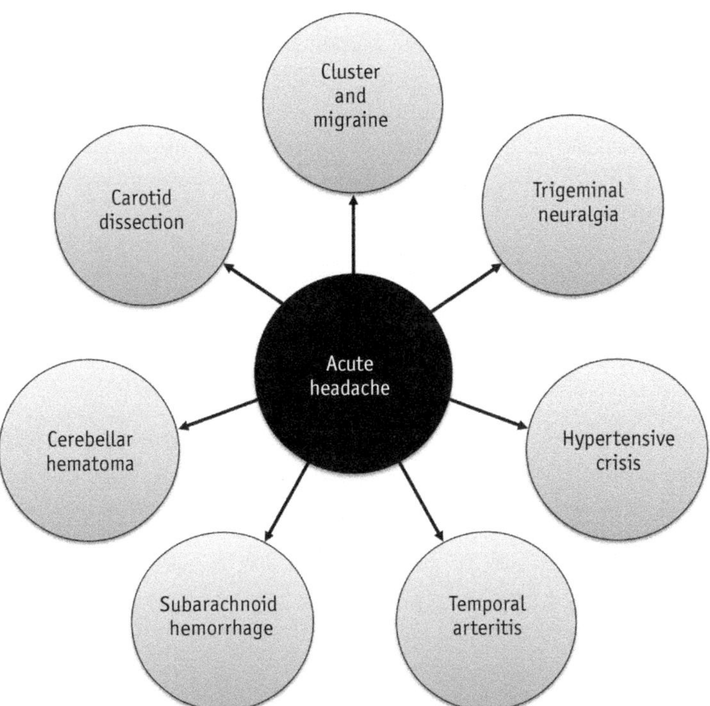

Figure 3.2 Common considerations in acute headache.

Table 3.1 **Unusual Neurologic Disorders Associated with Acute Headache**

- Cerebral venous thrombosis
- Pituitary apoplexy
- Cerebrospinal fluid hypovolemia syndrome
- Retroclival hematoma
- Reversible cerebral vasoconstriction syndrome
- Acute obstructive hydrocephalus from colloid cyst

A second common possible neurologic sign is vertigo. Neurologists see a fair number of these patients in the ED because balance is often off and patient may vomit and develop headache after prolonged vomiting. In evaluation of the dizzy patient, it is important to distinguish trigger mechanisms and timing of onset.

It remains a challenge for any specialist to reliably distinguish between a "central" of "peripheral" cause of vertigo. Acute onset versus a week's onset versus episodic onset, indicates a specific disorder in each. Any acute vestibular syndrome could indicate positional vertigo, a vestibular neuritis or posterior circulation stroke. Chronic vestibular syndromes are usually a result of drug effects or are functional. There are some important clues that point away from a cerebellar or brainstem lesion. Vomiting, sweating, pallor, tinnitus, and hearing loss are seen in vestibular lesions. Most emergency physicians are attuned to systemic triggers of vertigo, while neurologic examination is specifically focused on the brainstem and the type of nystagmus. Upbeat, downbeat, rebound, or dissociated nystagmus is often seen with central lesions in the upper and lower brainstem and cerebellum. Ocular bobbing—a downward jerk with slow return to midposition—is seen in a pontine lesion.

Ischemic stroke rarely presents with vertigo alone, but the combination of vertigo and gaze difficulty increases the probability of a stroke significantly. An important determinant of nystagmus is that a central nystagmus has direction dependence. When present, gaze toward the fast component of the nystagmus increases the frequency and amplitude. In central causes of nystagmus, gaze away from the direction of the fast component will achieve the opposite effect. Nystagmus that emerges with abrupt change in position and reduces with fixation also points to a peripheral lesion. Peripheral vestibular nystagmus can be muted by a visual fixation of the patient and would require Frenzel glasses. Positional nystagmus can also be demonstrated after a rapid change from sitting to head-hanging position. This maneuver, also known as the Dix-Hallpike maneuver, is a useful discriminatory test. The vestibuloocular reflex (quick head turn to one side by examiner) is abnormal when the patient cannot maintain eye fixation and indicates a peripheral lesion. Cooperation of the patient is key and may be suboptimal. Other testing of the vestibulospinal reflexes, including "past-pointing" or pointing beyond the examiner's finger in the finger-to-nose test, may not be discriminating enough. Static posture and tandem gait walking may evaluate vestibular function and cerebellar function, and unsteadiness and clumsiness (ataxia) can be seen with both peripheral and central lesions.[1,4,20]

One ED surveillance study[14] identified 1,273 dizziness cases (>45 years) and found a stroke in 2.2%. Moreover, 3 of 15 strokes had a stroke in cerebellum, brainstem, or thalamus. The study confirmed a common clinical impression of a largely nonstroke etiology for dizziness in the majority of presenting patients.[14] Considerations in acute vertigo are shown in Figure 3.3; neurologic disorders associated with acute vertigo are listed in Table 3.2.

The third major sign is syncope (Figure 3.4). Very few neurologic disorders are associated with syncope, but some should be considered (Table 3.3). Neurologists are not specifically asked to evaluate causes of syncope, just to exclude a seizure as a cause for syncope. Most often a neurologic consult is requested when a patient had "twitches" or had a somewhat prolonged recovery of consciousness. The evaluation of syncope is never complete in the ED. The cause of a single syncopal episode continues to be unknown in about a third of the patients and is usually due to neurally mediated syncope, such as a vasovagal attack, situational syncope, or carotid sinus syncope. In a not insignificant minority of patients is syncope symptomatic of a neurologic disorder. Generally, admission for diagnostic evaluation is mandatory for a patient with structural heart disease with symptoms suggestive of arrhythmia, ischemia, or electrocardiographic abnormalities. Frequently, patients are admitted for treatment of orthostatic hypotension or for evaluation of whether to discontinue or modify the use of a likely offending drug. Syncope in elderly persons can often be attributed to the use of antihypertensives, neuroleptics, tricyclic antidepressants, or dopaminergic agents and to some other trigger, such as dehydration. Syncope as a sign of acute occlusive vertebrobasilar disease is rare, but this potential cause is often a reason for consultation by a neurologist. Another principle is that most patients with syncope may have a systemic illness.[26–28]

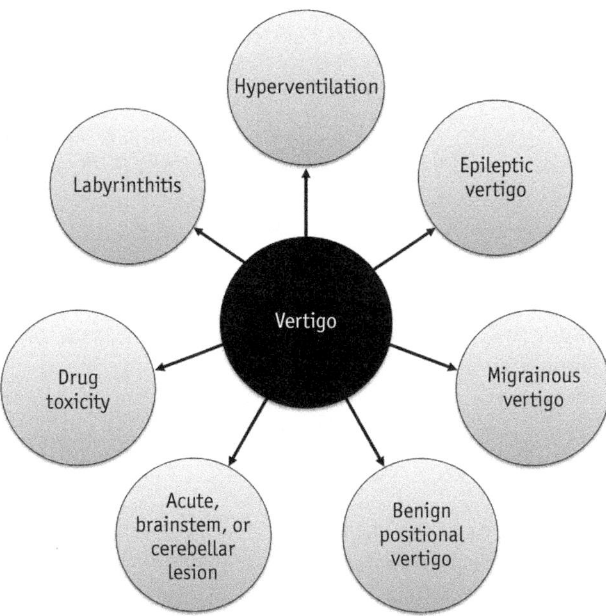

Figure 3.3 Common considerations in acute vertigo.

Table 3.2 **Specific Neurologic Disorders Associated with Acute Vertigo**

- Cerebellar stroke
- Thalamic infarct
- Acute vertebral artery occlusion
- Cerebellopontine tumor
- Acute MS plaque

History taking should include questions about the circumstances before the syncope attack, about the body position, and more—whether (1) the patient was supine, sitting, or standing; (2) the patient had symptoms at rest or with a change in posture; (3) the syncope occurred during urination, defecation, cough, or swallowing; and (4) predisposing factors were present (e.g., a crowded or warm environment, prolonged standing, or the immediate postprandial period).

Some syncope attacks are preceded by nausea, vomiting, abdominal discomfort, blurred vision, dizziness, and a feeling of cold sweat. Essential parts of history taking should also include such patient details as the way in which the patient fell (slumped or kneeled over), skin color, duration of loss of consciousness, breathing pattern and particularly loud breathing and snoring, movements and their duration, incontinence; and tongue biting.

Risk assessment is important in the ED. Several syncope rules have been developed; one of the most important is the San Francisco Syncope Rule.[24] The San Francisco Syncope Rule predictors are history of congestive heart failure, hematocrit less than 30%, abnormal electrocardiogram (EKG), complaint of shortness of breath,

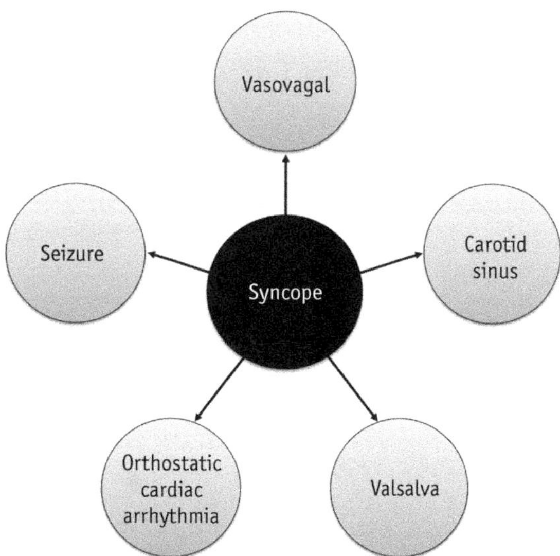

Figure 3.4 Common considerations in syncope.

Table 3.3 **Neurologic Disorders Associated with Syncope**

- Severe diabetic polyneuropathy
- Amyloid polyneuropathy
- Autoimmune autonomic neuropathy
- Olivopontocerebellar atrophy
- Shy–Drager syndrome
- Glossopharyngeal neuralgia
- Spinal cord injury

and systolic blood pressure less than 90 mm Hg during triage. In a validation study, the syncope rule had a sensitivity of 94%. Others have identified high-risk criteria such as a prior history of ventricular arrhythmias, cardiac device with dysfunction, exertional syncope, any presentations suggestive of acute coronary syndrome, prior severe cardiac valve disease, known poor ejection fraction, and abnormal EKG.[23,28] Other studies found that patients over 65 years old are four times more likely to have a cardiac syncope versus noncardiac syncope. Prior coronary artery disease or pathological Q waves also increase the odds of a cardiac syncope.[3]

The distinction between a seizure and a syncope is difficult to make (Chapter 6). During syncope, a standing person rarely falls down suddenly but often gradually slumps sideways; the person may have slurred speech followed by head nodding, eye closure, and loss of postural tone. Twitching and jerking and particularly myoclonus are often seen and these signs may be misinterpreted as seizures. Patients may be incontinent, which may simply reflect a full bladder at the time of the event. Pallor, a bitten tip of the tongue, and marked fatigue after the event may all be seen in syncope and do not prove an epileptic seizure. Typically, confusion that lasts more than 10 minutes, a lateral bite of the tongue, movement that is tonic and then clonic, and cyanosis are features of a seizure and may be helpful in differentiating syncope from a true seizure. Most seizures occur with no warning. By comparison, many patients with syncope recall that the "world was closing in" before they passed out. Seizures are most likely to be suspected when the patient had tonic–clonic movements that were witnessed. Inquiries about automatisms such as chewing, lip smacking, or frothing at the mouth, tongue biting, a blue instead of pale face, a funny or strange smell, prolonged confusion or even combativeness after the event may be useful and may point to a seizure rather than syncope. An important differentiating feature is that syncope which occurs during exercise is often cardiac in origin and may be related to volume depletion. Important elements in the history are the presence of nausea, sweating, and pallor, which indicate an autonomic component. Blurred vision and lightheadedness may also indicate autonomic failure. Syncope associated with dysautonomia can be related to patients who have a prior diabetes mellitus, parkinsonism, polyneuropathy, alcoholism, or recent start of blood-pressure-lowering medication.

In Practice

Although these are common presenting signs, their causes are not inexhaustibly numerous. Practically, it is useful to be aware of potential slip-ups with the evaluation of these mundane signs (Table 3.4).

There are several red flags in patients with acute headache. Any headache in an elderly patient (certainly if there is jaw claudication or visual loss) should be investigated with an erythrocyte sedimentation rate for temporal arteritis.[22] Any headache with fever requires a CSF and a CT scan for bacterial meningitis (or mastoiditis). Any headache with prior cancer could point to a new brain metastasis. Cerebral venous thrombosis may be considered if there is other evidence of thrombophilia and should be recognized in the postpartum period.[9] The best evaluation of patients with each of these symptoms results from close communication between the neurologist and the emergency physician. The emergency physician might assume the neurologist is able to identify a neurologic cause, and the neurologist might assume that the emergency room physician is able to identify a systemic cause. However, both should know the broad differential diagnosis of each of these symptoms. Sometimes, a neurologist—on his best and most memorable day—may diagnose acute glaucoma, temporal arteritis, and hypertensive emergency via a simple ophthalmoscopic examination. In acute glaucoma, the headache is associated with a red eye and a dilated pupil with poor light response; (it has been said that the affected eye also feels harder with palpation). Acute anterior ischemic optic neuropathy may be seen with marked disk

Table 3.4 **Potential Slip-ups**

Common Slip-ups in Acute Headache
• Assuming benign etiology after a response to drugs • Failure to describe and elaborate on thunderclap characteristic (new, different, 100% intense) • Failure to perform CT scan and lumbar puncture • Equating hemorrhagic CSF with SAH
Common Slip-ups in Vertigo
• Unreliable dizziness history • Poorly examined for gait difficulty • Poorly examined for nystagmus • Failure to look for vertical nystagmus, which is usually neurological
Common Slip-ups in Syncope
• Failure to recognize jerking movements before fall • Failure to recognize automatism • Failure to recognize tongue bite • Failure to recognize brainstem findings

CT = computed tomography; CSF = cerebrospinal fluid; SAH = subarachnoid hemorrhage swelling in the setting of giant cell arteritis. Acute papilledema with peripapillary flame-like hemorrhages or even a blood lake in the vitreous (Terson's syndrome) may point to a hypertensive emergency in a patient transferred with acute headache and (now) normal blood pressure from recent IV antihypertensive administration. Sometimes the emergency physician will be proud to have diagnosed carotid dissection by carefully listening for a carotid bruit in a young patient with a severe headache and a new Horner's syndrome.

Acute dizziness is usually not a stroke - if it is, gait instability is very common.[6] Nystagmus is generally not a useful clinical test to differentiate a central or peripheral cause in the ED, as there is wide overlap. Acute vertigo with deafness may indicate acute ischemic stroke in the cerebellum (superior cerebellar artery and anterior inferior cerebellar artery involvement) or a newly manifesting tumor in the cerebellopontine angle. Meniere's disease is very common, but recurrent attacks are usually seen with nausea and vomiting.

The most common type of syncope is vasovagal.[7,13,21] This syncope is caused by the inhibition of vasomotor centers in the medulla (e.g., due to compression of the carotid baroreceptors, emptying of a distended bladder or bowel, any overwhelming emotional shock), which causes bradycardia and vasodilatation. Orthostatic hypotension is suggested when syncope occurs after standing up, recent introduction of a medication that may lead to hypotension, in the presence of a neurodegenerative disease, or in the period after exertion. In younger persons, narcolepsy can be considered. Sudden loss of muscle tone (cataplexy) with laughing, anger, or an emotional response may cause these symptoms.

Risk stratification in the ED may be helpful for patients with syncope. A low-risk group (in which the syncope is likely benign) are patients younger than 50 years who have no previous history of cardiovascular disease, have normal cardiovascular examination, and have symptoms suggestive of a reflex-mediated or vasovagal syncope. Other patients may be admitted to a CCU for further evaluation of a possible cardiac arrhythmia.

During evaluation in the ED, specific attention is directed toward recognition of a long QT syndrome that mimics seizures, and interpretation errors are comparatively common. Holter monitoring is typically used for patients with syncope, but 24 hours may not be enough time for identifying potentially important arrhythmias. One study found that the diagnostic value of monitoring for evaluation of syncope was approximately 9%. Continuous-loop event monitoring may have increased yield, but its role has not been completely defined. An implantable continuous-loop recorder inserted subcutaneously has the capability of monitoring for about 18 months; however, the incidence of an event is low.

Simple measures that may be possible in the treatment of vasovagal syncope in an elderly person include physical countermaneuvers, salt supplementation, and use of fludrocortisone acetate and midodrine.

A final major problem in the ED is failure to do additional testing. Although the cost may significantly increase, many of us should err on the side of caution and proceed with neuroimaging, which may include imaging of the cerebral vasculature.[25]

Cost-effectiveness is complicated math in a litigious environment with demands for damages in the millions of dollars. Any patient with new brainstem findings or cerebellar findings should undergo an MRI scan. Any patient with a thunderclap headache should have a CT scan and possibly CTA before a decision is made on triage. Many CT scans of the brain are done for acute vertigo, and many are stone-cold normal, but a cerebellar lesion cannot be missed.

TRIAGE

Each of these disorders may have a different triage, some of which can be reasonably established in an emergency evaluation. Any patient with a thunderclap headache needs a CT scan of the brain and possibly a lumbar puncture, preferably by an experienced physician to avoid obtaining artificially blood-tinged CSF. Admission to an NICU is warranted in proven SAH, and a neurosurgical consultation is needed. Before the patient is transferred, it is advised to administer 1 g of tranexamic acid to reduce rebleeding while deciding on treatment. If no immediate cause of thunderclap headache is evident after testing, a decision can be made to transfer the patient to the ward.

The sensitivity of a plain CT scan of the brain in a patient with acute vertigo is very low. Also, an MRI is seldom acutely indicated in acute vertigo, unless a central type of nystagmus, cerebellar signs, facial asymmetry, or a new Horner's syndrome is found. An MRI is best combined with an MR angiogram if an ischemic stroke in the posterior fossa is considered. Still, many emergency physicians will send patients with acute vertigo home, often with drugs such as meclizine, scopolamine, or lorazepam.

It is urgent to admit and evaluate any patient with acute recurrent syncope to a monitored bed on the ward or CCU. An episode can then be closely observed and correlated to changes of blood pressure and heart rate. If none are found, more extensive neurologic testing may follow for primary neurologic disorders or 24-hour EEG monitoring may be performed to see whether seizures are the main culprit of bradycardia.

Putting It All Together

- Most thunderclap headaches indicate a serious event.
- Many headaches initially identified as thunderclap headaches turn out to have occurred far more gradually.
- Most acute dizziness in the ED is peripheral or systemic; it may rarely indicate a stroke, particularly a stroke in the posterior circulation.
- In the elderly, syncope is often caused by dehydration.
- In the young, syncope is often neurally mediated and emotion-related

By the Way

- Cardiac arrhythmias can cause syncope and mimic seizures.
- Neurologic examination is seldom helpful in acute headache and dizziness.
- Any new nystagmus requires urgent testing.
- Only a third of patients with severe headache may get a CT scan.

Acute Headache, Vertigo, and Syncope by the Numbers

- ~90% of patients with syncope have vasovagal syncope.
- ~50% of patients with acute dizziness may have a general medical cause.
- ~50% of patients with SAH had a warning headache but no investigation.
- ~20% of patients with their "worse headache ever" have CT scan abnormalities.
- ~10% of patients with acute headache may get a CSF examination.

References

1. Baloh RW, Honrubia V. *Clinical Neurophysiology of the Vestibular System* 3rd ed. New York: Oxford University Press; 2001.
2. Bellolio MF, Hess EP, Gilani WI, et al. External validation of the Ottowa subarachnoid hemorrhage clinical decision rule in patients with acute headache. *Am J Emerg Med* 2015;33:244–249.
3. Bhat PK, Pantham G, Laskey S, Como JJ, Rosenbaum DS. Recognizing cardiac syncope in patients presenting to the emergency department with trauma. *J Emerg Med* 2014;46:1–8.
4. Bronstein A, Lempert T. *Dizziness: A Practical Approach to Diagnosis and Management*. Cambridge: Cambridge University Press; 2007.
5. Bruce BB, Lamirel C, Wright DW, et al. Nonmydriatic ocular fundus photography in the emergency department. *N Engl J Med* 2011;364:387–389.
6. Chase M, Joyce NR, Carney E, et al. ED patients with vertigo: can we identify clinical factors associated with acute stroke? *Am J Emerg Med* 2012;30:587–591.
7. Chen LY, Benditt DG, Shen WK. Management of syncope in adults: an update. *Mayo Clin Proc* 2008;83:1280–1293.
8. Chu K, Hann A, Greenslade J, Williams J, Brown A. Spectrophotometry or visual inspection to most reliably detect xanthochromia in subarachnoid hemorrhage: systematic review. *Ann Emerg Med* 2014;64:256–264.
9. Cumurciuc R, Crassard I, Sarov M, Valade D, Bousser MG. Headache as the only neurological sign of cerebral venous thrombosis: a series of 17 cases. *J Neurol Neurosurg Psychiatry* 2005;76:1084–1087.
10. Czuczman AD, Thomas LE, Boulanger AB, et al. Interpreting red blood cells in lumbar puncture: distinguishing true subarachnoid hemorrhage from traumatic tap. *Acad Emerg Med* 2013;20:247–256.
11. Eskey CJ, Ogilvy CS. Fluoroscopy-guided lumbar puncture: decreased frequency of traumatic tap and implications for the assessment of CT-negative acute subarachnoid hemorrhage. *AJNR Am J Neuroradiol* 2001;22:571–576.
12. Goldstein JN, Camargo CA, Jr., Pelletier AJ, Edlow JA. Headache in United States emergency departments: demographics, work-up and frequency of pathological diagnoses. *Cephalalgia* 2006;26:684–690.
13. Kapoor WN. Syncope. *N Engl J Med* 2000;343:1856–1862.

14. Kerber KA, Zahuranec DB, Brown DL, et al. Stroke risk after nonstroke emergency department dizziness presentations: a population-based cohort study. *Ann Neurol* 2014;75:899–907.
15. Locker T, Mason S, Rigby A. Headache management—are we doing enough? An observational study of patients presenting with headache to the emergency department. *Emerg Med J* 2004;21:327–332.
16. Newman-Toker DE, Edlow JA. High-stakes diagnostic decision rules for serious disorders: the Ottawa subarachnoid hemorrhage rule. *JAMA* 2013;310:1237–1239.
17. Nicholl D, Weatherby S. Subarachnoid hemorrhage: the canary in the mine, or the elephant in the room? *Pract Neurol* 2014;14:204–205.
18. Perry JJ, Stiell IG, Sivilotti ML, et al. Clinical decision rules to rule out subarachnoid hemorrhage for acute headache. *JAMA* 2013;310:1248–1255.
19. Ramirez-Lassepas M, Espinosa CE, Cicero JJ, et al. Predictors of intracranial pathologic findings in patients who seek emergency care because of headache. *Arch Neurol* 1997;54:1506–1509.
20. Seemungal BM, Bronstein AM. A practical approach to acute vertigo. *Pract Neurol* 2008;8:211–221.
21. Smars PA, Decker WW, Shen WK. Syncope evaluation in the emergency department. *Curr Opin Cardiol* 2007;22:44–48.
22. Smetana GW, Shmerling RH. Does this patient have temporal arteritis? *JAMA* 2002;287:92–101.
23. Sun BC, McCreath H, Liang LJ, et al. Randomized clinical trial of an emergency department observation syncope protocol versus routine inpatient admission. *Ann Emerg Med* 2014;64:167–175.
24. Tan C, Sim TB, Thng SY. Validation of the San Francisco Syncope Rule in two hospital emergency departments in an Asian population. *Acad Emerg Med* 2013;20:487–497.
25. Ward MJ, Bonomo JB, Adeoye O, Raja AS, Pines JM. Cost-effectiveness of diagnostic strategies for evaluation of suspected subarachnoid hemorrhage in the emergency department. *Acad Emerg Med* 2012;19:1134–1144.
26. Wieling W, Krediet CT, Wilde AA. Flush after syncope: not always an arrhythmia. *J Cardiovasc Electrophysiol* 2006;17:804–805.
27. Wiener Z, Chiu DT, Shapiro NI, Grossman SA. Substance abuse in emergency department patients with unexplained syncope. *Intern Emerg Med* 2014;9:331–334.
28. Wilk JS, Nardone AL, Jennings CA, Crausman RS. Unexplained syncope: when to suspect pulmonary thromboembolism. *Geriatrics* 1995;50:46–50.

4

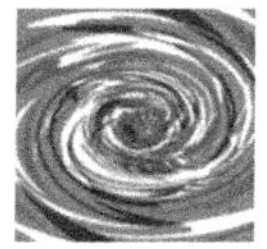

Treating Acute Neurologic Pain Syndromes

Acute pain motivates patients to visit an ED or even call 911. Intense acute or prolonged severe unremitting pain is a common reason to rush to the ED; depending on other symptomatology, some patients may be critical. Sadly, patients with acute-on-chronic pain may populate EDs asking for relief with narcotics—and often get it. The maladies of these patients and their perception of undertreatment are well known to emergency physicians, but most feel the ED is not the right place for them and is misused for "opioid shopping."

But there are other patients who visit the ED whose pain is acutely serious. Acute pain in abdomen and chest is common in the ED, but neurologic causes are not often considered, and it may only be after no other systemic illness has been found that a neurological basis for the patient's complaint is sought. There are several quite characteristic neurologic pain syndromes.

Acute pain of neurologic origin is often an emergency and needs to be taken seriously. Effective pain management remains difficult in the ED. This chapter discusses the appropriate selection and dosing of drugs to treat severe acute pain associated with acute neurologic diseases. The most important questions are as follows: How can we best characterize neurologic pain? What pain syndromes are particularly challenging? What are the essential tests in the ED to diagnose the source of acute pain?

This chapter provides a guide to the management of acute neurologic causes of pain that need to be triaged appropriately. Neuropathic pain can be caused by metabolic disorder (diabetes mellitus, vitamin B deficiency), infections (varicella zoster, HIV), toxins (chemotherapy), and injuries (trauma or entrapment).[34] When it comes to acute pain signaling an emergency, an accurate and pointed history is all that counts.

Principles

One of the first core principle is to define the different types of pain. Neuropathic pain may be burning, lancinating, or electrical. Pain may increase after repetitive stimulation, and pain may occur with a stimulus that normally does not evoke pain (known as allodynia). A stimulus that causes exaggerated pain is also neuropathic (known as hyperalgesia). In any new lesions (nerve, spinal cord, thalamus), there is a general sense that the appearance of hypersensitivity predates persistent pain.[20,21,34] Examination is with simple techniques (Table 4.1), but mapping of an affected area may require close patient cooperation and a considerable amount of patience. A pin can produce allodynia, hyperalgesia, or nothing.

The second core principle is that neuropathic pain is a combination of numbness, pain with a mild stimulus such as touch of the skin or electric and shock-like. Sorting out the specific sensations may help in possible localization. Patients with peripheral neuropathies may complain of tingling or burning, prickling, tightness, shooting (lancinating) pain, and the feeling of walking on stones. When small fibers are involved (diabetes, amyloid angiopathy, hereditary neuropathies), the symptoms are more aching, burning, and tingling. Causalgia is burning pain in a peripheral nerve distribution. Spinal cord lesions produce band tightness (lemniscal tracts), and nerve root involvement produces shooting pain (sciatica).

Central neuropathic pain is related to a lesion in the spinal cord or brain. Spinal cord injury pain is usually below or at the level of the injury. Central pain originating from the brain often follows a stroke or a neurosurgical resection. Most patients have spontaneous dysesthesias (abnormal sense of touch), and patients may describe cutting, squeezing, and tearing pain. The lesion responsible is the thalamus, but "thalamic pain" has also been associated with other localizations such as cortex, operculum, and lateral medulla.[16]

Pain associated with avulsion of nerves can cause excruciating deafferentation pain—the most known is avulsion of the brachial plexus. Pain occurs usually years later. These types of pain can be continuous, often burning or throbbing (assumed to be due to thalamic neuroplasticity), or shooting paroxysms (assumed to be due to dorsal horn hyperactivity). The ventroposterolateral nucleus of the sensory thalamus

Table 4.1 **Assessment of Pain**

- Mapping areas of allodynia, hyperalgesia, hypoalgesia, and anesthesia
- Cotton ball, pinprick
- Finger pressure
- Fingers squeeze
- Cold (any metal object)
- Hot (warm water tube)

rather than periventricular gray is the first target of choice for deep brain stimulation to relieve this limb pain.

The third core principle is that acute neurologic pain may be the only symptom without any other pointers on clinical examination. Pain is just there and nothing can be observed other than a markedly distressed or uncomfortable patient. (It is different with abdominal pain, where prodding may elicit the pain, or even chest pain, where patients have EKG abnormalities or are tachypneic or tachycardic). A good example is acute face or ear pain in the setting of herpes zoster infection.[35] Patients may have severe excruciating pain in that area without any clear abnormal skin lesions, which may appear later. These lesions are usually erythematous and maculopapular, and may even appear 24–48 hours after the severe onset of pain. Herpes zoster infection may involve severe facial pain, photophobia, and malaise; it may last for up to 5 days before appearance of vesicles. Another good example is severe shoulder pain that is not associated with any neurologic symptoms, but a result of an autoimmune brachioplexitis (Parsonage–Turner syndrome). These patients may have severe shoulder pain that may last for days to even weeks—pain that is often sharp and stabbing and may even suggest an acute radiculopathy—but nothing out of the ordinary is found on examination, sometimes not even muscle weakness. These symptoms occur later and may progress rapidly. Another known example is that epidural hematoma or epidural abscess may present with severe low back pain without any clear neurologic findings suggesting an evolving myelopathy. Most of the neurologic findings do appear shortly after the acute onset, but emergency physicians and neurologists may be deceived by the absence of any objective findings.

The fourth core principle is that in any acute neurologic pain syndrome, adequate pain management is feasible, effective, and simple, but most patients have been poorly managed.[8] Inadequate pain management in acute neurologic pain syndromes is usually due to unfamiliarity with the available drugs and underdosing. Unfamiliarity with newer agents is also a factor because the pharmacopeia of pain management is continuously growing and changing. Tricyclic antidepressants and antiepileptic drugs found their way in pain treatment, and now drugs that target NMDA receptors, cannabinoid receptors, and tumor necrosis factor-alpha (TNF-α)—among many others—are in development.

To understand pain management is to understand how drugs could alleviate pain. Some drugs, such as carbamazepine and lidocaine, act on membrane excitability. Baclofen and midazolam act on the synapse and the gamma-aminobutyric acid (GABA) receptor. Antidepressants (both tricyclic antidepressants and serotonin-norepinephrine reuptake inhibitors [amitriptyline, trazodone, duloxetine]) suppress ectopic firing. None of these drugs are "rescue" drugs and their effect is protracted. Opioids are therefore often simultaneously prescribed with relentless pain (Table 4.2).

A fourth principle is to define and measure adequate pain control. This is an area of contention because of its profound subjectivity. Most clinicians use a visual analog scale. Patients mark the line that goes from no relief of pain to complete relief of pain or, when it pertains to intensity, from no pain to worst pain. The patient will need to remember the intensity of the pain to assess the degree

Table 4.2 **Commonly Used Medications for Treating Neuropathic Pain**

Pharmacological Mechanism	*Drug (class)*	*Dosing (mg)*		
		Starting	*Maintenance*	*Frequency*
Sodium channel blockade	Topical lidocaine (5%)	1–4 patches	1–4 patches	12 h on
Serotonin, norepinephrine reuptake inhibition, sodium channel blockade	Amitriptyline (antidepressant—tertiary amine tricyclic)	10–25	50–150	Once daily at nighttime
	Nortriptyline (antidepressant—secondary amine tricyclic)	10–25	50–100	Once daily at nighttime
Selective serotonin reuptake inhibition	Paroxetine	10–20	20–80	Once daily in the morning
	Citalopram	10–20	20–80	Once daily in the morning
Serotonin, norepinephrine reuptake inhibition	Duloxetine	20–30	60	Once or twice daily
Selective serotonin, norepinephrine reuptake inhibition	Venlafaxine	37.5–50.0	150–300	Once daily in the morning
Dopamine, norepinephrine reuptake inhibition	Bupropion	50–100	200–400	Once daily in the morning
Calcium channel antagonism	Gabapentin	100–300	900–3,600	Divided 3 times daily
Sodium channel blockade	Carbamazepine	100–200	600–1,200	Divided twice daily
Sodium channel blockade, glutamate release inhibition	Lamotrigine	25–50	300–500	Divided twice daily
Calcium channel antagonism	Pregabalin	50–100	150–600	3 times daily
Opioid μ-receptor agonist	Oxycodone	5–10	20–160	Every 4–6 h
	Morphine	15–30	30–300	Every 4–6 h
	Transdermal fentanyl	25 μg/h patch	25–150 μg/h patch	Every 48–72 h

(continued)

Table 4.2 **Continued**

Pharmacological Mechanism	*Drug (class)*	*Dosing (mg)*		
		Starting	*Maintenance*	*Frequency*
Opioid μ-receptor agonist, NMDA receptor antagonism	Methadone	5–10	20–80	1–4 times daily
Nonopioid μ-receptor agonist, serotonin, norepinephrine reuptake inhibition	Tramadol	37.5–50.0	200–400	Every 6–8 h

Note: NMDA = *N*-methyl-D-aspartate.

Source: Pain Medicine: An Interdisciplinary Case-Based Approach. Oxford University Press (Hayek, Shah, & Desai, 2015).

of relief. Most pain experts and patients have considered 50% relief from maximum pain as clinically relevant.

In Practice

It is crucial to relieve pain in the ED after the diagnosis is established. Common reasons for neurologic pain consultation in the ED are shown in Figure 4.1. Here we systematically approach the problem by key symptom presentation and proceed with best initial management. The ED is not the place for prolonged observation of patients with pain as a result of an evolving neurologic disease, and admission is often clearly indicated.

ACUTE HEADACHE SYNDROME

Most patients in the ED present with an exacerbation of chronic migraine. This will have to be differentiated from a thunderclap headache, where the patient has an acute split-second headache that is out of the ordinary and not recognized by the patient despite a prior headache history—it often feels as if the head is blown off. Some patients may lose consciousness at the onset; those patients require a CT scan and a lumbar puncture, and often a CTA initially to look for a ruptured intracranial aneurysm.[31] (Further detailed discussion is found in Chapter 3.) Most acute migraine attacks present fairly rapidly, within a matter of hours, and are often too painful for the patient to handle at home. In most instances, patients have tried at least one drug without having relief, sometimes even two, before a trip is considered to the ED.

The management for migraine status is multifaceted and involves the use of opioids, antidopaminergic agents, and NSAIDs, among other agents. Most headache experts feel that acute migraine is best managed with an oral or nasal therapy with a triptan or

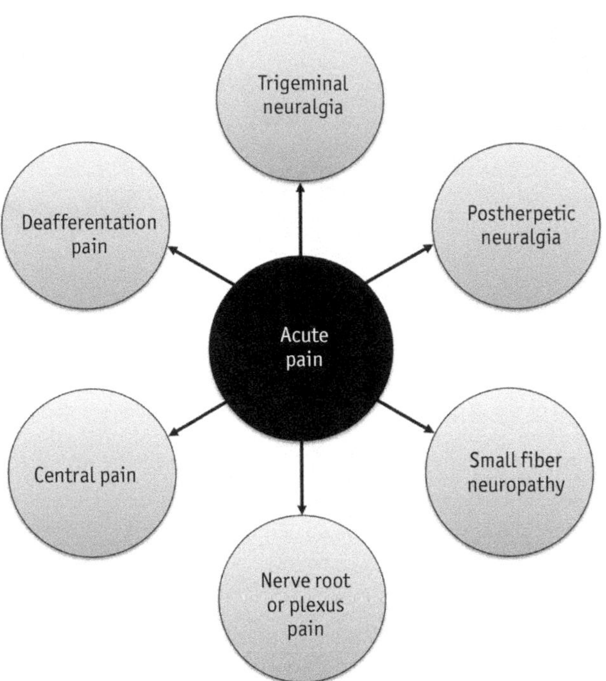

Figure 4.1 Causes of acute neuropathic pain in the emergency department.

NSAID,[2] and ketorolac appears to be an effective agent for relief of acute migraine headache.[32] Other options are oral naproxen, using 500 mg twice a day. Contraindications for use of triptans include familial hemiplegic migraine, ischemic stroke, ischemic heart disease, Prinzmetal's angina, uncontrolled hypertension, combination with monoamine oxidase inhibitors or ergot compounds, and pregnancy. In many EDs, corticosteroids for status migrainosis have been administered, often involving the use of dexamethasone. There is no evidence that a corticosteroid course impacts on initial management or prevention of recurrence. Recent recommendations have been published by the American Headache Society.[26] Some of the options are show in Table 4.3.

Dopamine receptor antagonists such as chlorpromazine or prochlorperazine are other agents that should be additionally administered if the patient is nauseated.[7] With severe nausea, dehydration follows rapidly, so IV fluids need to be administered. A recent study found that IV sodium valproate was ineffective and inferior to metoclopramide or ketorolac.[15,17] In a large double-blind study randomizing patients to 10 mg of metoclopramide or 30 mg of ketorolac administered as an IV drip over 15 minutes, headache freedom was achieved in 11% of metoclopramide patients and 16% of the patients with ketorolac. Relief was much lower with use of valproate, where only 4% improvement was noted. Most notable is that these drugs only help a small proportion of patients, suggesting that other drugs might be necessary.

Currently, the use of dihydroergotamine (DHE) or subcutaneous sumatriptan followed by parenteral NSAIDs is considered a reasonable initial option in acute migraine. Best studies remain with sumatriptan 6 mg by subcutaneous

Table 4.3 **US Trade Names for Generic Drugs Used in Emergency Room Management of Acute Migraine**

Class of Medication	*Generic Drug Name*
Opioids	Meperidine
Dopamine-receptor antagonists	Chlorpromazine Prochlorperazine Promethazine Droperidol Haloperidol Metoclopramide
Triptans	Sumatriptan Zolmitriptan
NSAIDs	Ketorolac Diclofenac
Corticosteroids	Dexamethasone
Antiepileptics	Sodium valproate

Source: From Gelfand and Goadsby.[17]

injection; however, this is much less effective if the headache has exceeded 6 hours.[2] Another option is to use DHE 0.5–1 mg in IV or IM dose repeated to maximum of 3 mg in 24 hours. Nausea is much less with the intramuscular dose of DHE.[17] The response of cluster headache to subcutaneous sumatriptan or oxygen by nasal cannula is excellent. Intranasal lidocaine or zolmitriptan are good abortive therapies. Abortive treatments for patients with "therapy-resistant, persistent" headache lasting for hours are shown in Table 4.4.

An acute headache in a patient who is pregnant or postpartum is quite common, but most have a tension-type headache—few have preeclampsia or migraine exacerbation. Some of these patients may have a postpartum exacerbation of migraine that has improved during pregnancy. Patients with low-pressure headaches may start to develop these headaches several days after delivery and epidural analgesia and during mobilization, with immediate resolution upon lying flat. The treatment is usually a blood patching and is successful.

ACUTE EYE AND FACE PAIN

Acute eye pain associated with acute diplopia is also known as the painful ophthalmoplegias. In these patients, there may be a combination of third nerve palsy, acute sixth nerve palsy, or acute fourth nerve palsy.[3,9,23–25] Patients with a ruptured posterior communicating cerebral artery aneurysm, mucormycosis, cavernous sinus thrombosis, meningitis, or herpes zoster ophthalmicus can all present with acute diplopia and a cranial nerve deficit. Acute oculomotor palsy with retro-orbital pain might be a sign of an enlarging or dissecting posterior communicating cerebral artery

Table 4.4 **Abortive Therapies for Acute Head and Face Pain**

Disorder	*Therapy Options*
Migraine	• Sumatriptan 20 mg nasal spray or Sumatriptan 6 mg SC; repeat after 1 hour, if needed • Droperidol (2.75–8.25 mg IM) • Meperidine (100 mg IM) and hydroxyzine (50 mg IM) • Valproate sodium (1,000 mg IV in 50 mL normal saline over 5 minutes) • Dihydroergotamine (1–3 mg IV at hourly intervals) and metoclopramide (10 mg IM) • Ketorolac 30–60 mg IM
Cluster headache	• Oxygen therapy (7 L/min facemask) • Metoclopramide (10 mg IM) • Sumatriptan (6 mg SC) • Nasal butorphanol (1 mg/1 puff) • Intranasal lidocaine 4% (4 sprays)
Trigeminal neuralgia	• Fosphenytoin (15–20 mg/kg IV) • Lamotrigine (50–100 mg/day) • Topiramate (50–100 mg/day)

SC = subcutaneous; IM = intramuscular; IV = intravenous.

aneurysm—rupture may occur within 24–48 hours after presentation. New pupil involvement and anisocoria indicates an immediate need for cerebral angiogram.

Acute face pain may be related to acute onset of trigeminal neuralgia or herpes zoster ophthalmicus.[18] Typically, there is periorbital reddening and edema with erythematous vesicles in V1 and V2 regions within 24 hours.[4,35] Therefore, the recognition can be very difficult early on, but excruciating pain and severe discomfort could point in this direction. There are specific emergency room treatments that can help in aborting the pain. In patients with trigeminal neuralgia, fosphenytoin loading with 20 mg/kg IV or the use of lamotrigine or topiramate can be abortive in a patient who has severe, unrelenting jabs of facial pain that are typically triggered by facial touch, chewing, or even talking. Spray of 8% lidocaine may help in some patients.[36] If herpes zoster ophthalmicus is diagnosed, the patient should be immediately treated with oral acyclovir 800 mg five times daily, usually within 24 hours of lesion onset. Escalating doses of gabapentin can be helpful early. Amitriptyline is better for postherpetic pain.[5] An alternative option is valacyclovir, which is superior to acyclovir when it relates to improvement of zoster-associated pain.[4] In many instances, the use of oxycodone or any other long-acting opioid preparations might be useful to treat the initial pain episodes, which can be severe and nocturnal. The use of tricyclic antidepressants or gabapentin can be considered; however, it would take several days for these drugs to be effective. Again, gabapentin significantly reduces postherpatic neuralgia, usually starting with a dose of 300 mg three times a day and increasing to 2,400 mg daily. Pregabalin 50–75 mg twice day up to 600 mg/day is tolerated by many patients as long as the increase is weekly. Topical application of capsaicin is not useful.[22]

ACUTE SHOULDER AND ARM PAIN

High intensity neck and upper extremity pain, and major disability from limitation in almost all daily activities will bring a patient to the ED. Most common causes of cervical radiculopathy are disc protrusion, cervical spondylosis, and cervical spinal stenosis. Inflammatory mechanisms other than mechanical compression have been proposed ("chemical radiculitis"). The diagnosis of acute radiculopathy is rarely confirmed on examination. It remains difficult to differentiate it from tendinitis or capsulitis. Many of these patients have significant pain that has emerged rapidly and is shooting, radiating in arm or fingers. Characteristically, patients do not initially have any numbness or weakness or any other associated symptoms. Usually, there is a pins-and-needles sensation or burning, but the transient is sharp, and nerve root pain is commonly worsened with Valsalva maneuvers or certain positioning changes. Severe shoulder pain with no clear abnormalities on examination could point toward an autoimmune plexitis in which the pain may last for several weeks—sharp, stabbing, and throbbing—and involves the neck and arm followed by muscle weakness only weeks after the pain has started and which may even occur when the pain is subsiding. The weakness becomes profound, often involving proximal muscles, causing scapular winging and significant atrophy of hand and proximal muscles. Commonly affected muscles are the infraspinatus, supraspinatus, deltoid, serratus anterior, biceps, and triceps. Some patients may have more distal abnormalities.[30]

The so-called upper limb tension test A is most sensitive for cervical radiculopathy and is considered the "straight-leg raise test" of the upper extremity. The test is to sequentially perform the following movements: scapular depression, shoulder abduction, forearm supination, wrist and finger extension, shoulder lateral rotation, elbow extension, and contralateral cervical side bending. The commonly performed Spurling test is less sensitive and involves passively side-bending the neck to the symptomatic side while putting downward pressure on the patient's head. The extension of the neck usually exacerbates a cervical radiculopathy and of course does not exacerbate acute plexitis. Radiographic imaging is necessary and MRI scan of the neck might be useful to exclude a compressive lesion. The common radiculopathies are shown in Table 4.5.

The natural course of cervical radiculopathy is not exactly known. Clinical experience has taught that about a third of the patients are pain- and symptom-free after several months, one-third may have mild and nondisabling symptoms and no clear identifiable signs, and one-third progress or have persistent pain in need of some sort of surgical intervention. Some studies have reported an even more favorable course average at the 6 month benchmark. Nerve conduction studies are a useful test for evaluating for radiculopathy, but only after several weeks' duration of pain. Many early radiculopathies may have a sensory and demyelinating component. The EMG portion of the study can point to a certain root level and provide some information on the acuteness of the radiculopathy.

Treatment of acute radiculopathies is medical, initially using physical therapy protocols and adequate pain management with anti-inflammatory agents; if it persists, interventional pain management and surgical management are considered. Multiple pharmacologic agents, immobilization with a collar, physical therapy, manipulation,

Table 4.5 **Findings in Common Radiculopathies**

Disc	*Root*	*Pain/Dysesthesias*	*Sensory Loss*	*Weakness*	*Reflex Loss*
C4-5	C5	Neck, shoulder, upper arm	Shoulder	Deltoid, biceps, infraspinatus	Biceps
C5-6	C6	Neck, shoulder, lateral arm, radial forearm, thumb, index finger	Lateral arm, radial forearm, thumb, index finger	Biceps, brachioradialis, supinator	Biceps, brachioradialis
C6-7	C7	Neck, lateral arm, ring through index fingers	Radial forearm, index and middle fingers	Triceps, extensor carpi ulnaris	Triceps
C7-T1	C8	Ulnar forearm and hand	Ulnar half or ring finger, little finger	Intrinsic hand muscles, wrist extensors, flexor digitorum profundus	Finger flexion
L3-4	L4	Anterior thigh, inner shin	Anteromedial thigh and shin, inner foot	Quadriceps	Patella
L4-5	L5	Lateral thigh and calf, dorsum of foot, great toe	Lateral calf and great toe	Extensor hallices longus, ± foot dorsiflexion, inversion and eversion	None
L5-S1	S1	Back of thigh, lateral posterior calf, lateral foot	Posterolateral calf, lateral and sole of foot, smaller toes	Gastrocnemius ± foot eversion	Achilles

Source: From Goldstein and Greer.[19]

traction, and transcutaneous electrical nerve stimulation have all been used in the treatment of cervical radiculopathy, with more claims of success than hard data. A collar is no more effective than physiotherapy, and traction may not be more effective than placebo. Surgery is considered for patients with intractable symptoms and signs of radiculopathy or a major motor deficit. As expected, the evidence for cervical transforaminal epidural injections is marginal; controlled trials comparing interlaminar epidural injections with local anesthetic and corticosteroids or local anesthetic may be needed. Such a trial would also carefully register complications (e.g., infections). Brainstem stroke or cervical spinal cord infarcts after accidental artery injection reportedly occur in less than 1% of injections.

ACUTE BACK PAIN

Obviously, acute back pain is a common complaint in patients seen in the ED, but it is potentially concerning.[10,12–14,19] The most important red flags in patients who have acute back pain are: pain lasting more than 6 weeks, prior history of cancer, the presence of fever or increased white blood cell count, a recent bacterial infection or injection, and possible trauma. Acute back pain may radiate to the buttocks or to the thigh, but typically also past the knee. The pain increases with movement, and on physical examination, the specific L4-S1 nerve roots are specifically investigated. This includes an examination of the sensory anatomy as well as reflexes and strength level. However, the sensitivity of sensory examination in the diagnosis of acute radiculopathy is low, probably not more than 25%. Bladder, bowel, and saddle sensory changes are predictive factors for compression and there is a higher likelihood of cord or cauda compression. Most important is to investigate abnormal perianal sensation (S3-S5) and rectal tone (S2-S5). Bladder function becomes impaired if the nerve roots S1-S4 are involved. The straight-leg-raising test has an 90% sensitivity for an acute herniated disc, but only if this produces radicular pain below the knee.[29] Pain increases on sudden dorsiflexion of the foot. (Braggart sign). Acute back pain may indicate a lumbar-sacral disc disease or radiculopathy but also occasionally epidural abscess or epidural hematoma, usually with more significant development of neurologic symptoms and spinal cord compression.[11] Many of these patients rapidly develop cauda equina symptomatology, in which case immediate testing with MRI and possible surgical intervention is necessary. (Further details are in Chapter 9 on triaging CNS infections.)

Surgical management of most lumbosacral radiculopathies is based on severity of pain and weakness.[1,6] Pain control for acute radicular low back pain is difficult; and responds best to ketorolac but not IV lidocaine.[33] IV methylprednisolone does not improve pain control.

Cauda equina syndrome may present in the ED. Late recognition and thus late surgery will result in bladder control problems. The main issue is that only in approximately 1 in 100 cases of disc herniation, an advanced cauda syndrome is seen. Generally, urodynamic studies are better in patients treated earlier, but surgery before or after 48 hours did not impact on need for intermittent catheterization.[28] Studies are difficult to interpret due to differences in techniques (e.g., wide laminectomies) and preoperative neurologic examination.

TRIAGE

Certain acute pain syndromes are emergencies that require immediate and multidisciplinary evaluation. The word “immediate” is key here. Some patients may need to be seen by a neurosurgeon for further testing and even same-day surgery. Some patients need immediate pain control and proof of relief after observation in the ED.

Putting It All Together

- Neuropathic pain is characterized by positive and negative symptoms.
- Pain may have no other clinical findings; some may appear later.
- Pain control for most acute neuropathic syndromes is possible using medication, often in combination.
- Acute surgery for refractory pain is seldom indicated.
- Cauda equina compression presents with back pain, weakness, and acute urinary retention (in combination).

By the Way

- There are considerable drug interactions with aggressive pain control.
- Calming the patient may be necessary.
- Adequate pain control still requires immediate evaluation for the cause of pain.
- Difficulty achieving pain control is often a result of undertreatment.

Acute Neurologic Pain by the Numbers

- ~95% of patients with trigeminal neuralgia have vascular compression.
- ~70% of patients with trigeminal neuralgia have touch-induced allodynia.
- ~30% of patients with neuropathic pain respond to first-line treatment.
- ~25% of brachial plexus avulsions have deafferentation pain.
- ~20% of patients with chronic pain may suffer from neuropathic pain.
- ~4% trigeminal neuralgia recur after decompressive surgery.

References

1. Ahn UM, Ahn NU, Buchowski JM, et al. Cauda equina syndrome secondary to lumbar disc herniation: a meta-analysis of surgical outcomes. *Spine* 2000;25:1515–1522.
2. Akpunonu BE, Mutgi AB, Federman DJ, et al. Subcutaneous sumatriptan for treatment of acute migraine in patients admitted to the emergency department: a multicenter study. *Ann Emerg Med* 1995;25:464–469.
3. Anagnostou E, Kouzi I, Kararizou E. Painful ophthalmoplegia: the role of imaging and steroid response in the acute and subacute setting. *J Neurol Sci* 2013;331:145–149.
4. Beutner KR, Friedman DJ, Forszpaniak C, Andersen PL, Wood MJ. Valaciclovir compared with acyclovir for improved therapy for herpes zoster in immunocompetent adults. *Antimicrob Agents Chemother* 1995;39:1546–1553.
5. Bowsher D. The effects of pre-emptive treatment of postherpetic neuralgia with amitriptyline: a randomized, double-blind, placebo-controlled trial. *J Pain Symptom Manage* 1997;13:327–331.
6. Bruggeman AJ, Decker RC. Surgical treatment and outcomes of lumbar radiculopathy. *Phys Med Rehabil Clin N Am* 2011;22:161–177.
7. Charbit AR, Akerman S, Goadsby PJ. Dopamine: what's new in migraine? *Curr Opin Neurol* 2010;23:275–281.

8. Chen H, Lamer TJ, Rho RH, et al. Contemporary management of neuropathic pain for the primary care physician. *Mayo Clin Proc* 2004;79:1533–1545.
9. Chou KL, Galetta SL, Liu GT, et al. Acute ocular motor mononeuropathies: prospective study of the roles of neuroimaging and clinical assessment. *J Neurol Sci* 2004;219:35–39.
10. Corwell BN. The emergency department evaluation, management, and treatment of back pain. *Emerg Med Clin North Am* 2010;28:811–839.
11. Darouiche RO. Spinal epidural abscess. *N Engl J Med* 2006;355:2012–2020.
12. Della-Giustina DA. Emergency department evaluation and treatment of back pain. *Emerg Med Clin North Am* 1999;17:877–893, vi–vii.
13. Deyo RA, Rainville J, Kent DL. What can the history and physical examination tell us about low back pain? *JAMA* 1992;268:760–765.
14. Deyo RA, Weinstein JN. Low back pain. *N Engl J Med* 2001;344:363–370.
15. Friedman BW, Garber L, Yoon A, et al. Randomized trial of IV valproate vs metoclopramide vs ketorolac for acute migraine. *Neurology* 2014;82:976–983.
16. Garcia-Larrea L, Perchet C, Creac'h C, et al. Operculo-insular pain (parasylvian pain): a distinct central pain syndrome. *Brain* 2010;133:2528–2539.
17. Gelfand AA, Goadsby PJ. A neurologist's guide to acute migraine therapy in the emergency room. *Neurohospitalist* 2012;2:51–59.
18. Gershon AA, Perkin RT. Herpes zoster. *N Engl J Med* 2000;343:222.
19. Goldstein JN, Greer DM. Rapid focused neurological assessment in the emergency department and ICU. *Emerg Med Clin North Am* 2009;27:1–16.
20. Jensen TS, Baron R, Haanpaa M, et al. A new definition of neuropathic pain. *Pain* 2011;152:2204–2205.
21. Jensen TS, Finnerup NB. Allodynia and hyperalgesia in neuropathic pain: clinical manifestations and mechanisms. *Lancet Neurol* 2014;13:924–935.
22. Johnson RW, Rice AS. Clinical practice. Postherpetic neuralgia. *N Engl J Med* 2014;16;371:1526–1533.
23. Keane JR. Bilateral sixth nerve palsy: analysis of 125 cases. *Arch Neurol* 1976;33:681–683.
24. Keane JR. Fourth nerve palsy: historical review and study of 215 inpatients. *Neurology* 1993;43:2439–2443.
25. Keane JR. Third nerve palsy: analysis of 1400 personally-examined inpatients. *Can J Neurol Sci* 2010;37:662–670.
26. Marmura MJ, Silberstein SD, Schwedt TJ. The acute treatment of migraine in adults: the American headache society evidence assessment of migraine pharmacotherapies. *Headache* 2015;55:3–20.
27. Morris EW, Di Paola M, Vallance R, Waddell G. Diagnosis and decision making in lumbar disc prolapse and nerve entrapment. *Spine* 1986;11:436–439.
28. Olivero WC, Wang H, Hanigan WC, et al. Cauda equina syndrome (CES) from lumbar disc herniations. *J Spinal Disord Tech* 2009;22:202–206.
29. Ropper AH, Zafonte RD. Sciatica. *N Engl J Med* 2015;372:1240–1248.
30. Smith CC, Bevelaqua AC. Challenging pain syndromes: Parsonage-Turner syndrome. *Phys Med Rehabil Clin N Am* 2014;25:265–277.
31. Stewart H, Reuben A, McDonald J. LP or not LP, that is the question: gold standard or unnecessary procedure in subarachnoic hemorrhage? *EMJ* 2014;31:720–7230.
32. Taggart E, Doran S, Kokotillo A, et al. Ketorolac in the treatment of acute migraine: a systematic review. *Headache* 2013;53:277–287.
33. Tanen DA, Shimada M, Danish DC, et al. Intravenous lidocaine for the emergency department treatment of acute radicular low back pain, a randomized controlled trial. *J Emerg Med* 2014;47:119–124.
34. von Hehn CA, Baron R, Woolf CJ. Deconstructing the neuropathic pain phenotype to reveal neural mechanisms. *Neuron* 2012;73:638–652.
35. Wijdicks EFM, Win PH. Excrutiating headache but nothing obvious, look at the skin! *Pract Neurol* 2004;4:302–303.
36. Zakrzewska JM, Linskey ME. Trigeminal neuralgia. *BMJ* 2014;348:g474.

5

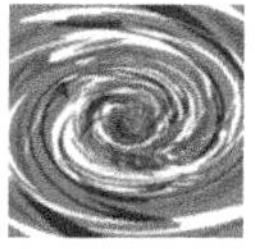

Treating Movement Disorder Emergencies

It would be a fair statement that correct diagnosis of a movement disorder is a difficult task and that the seriousness of an acute movement disorder is underappreciated. Any wildly "flailing and shaking" patient catches attention, but acute immobility from hypokinesis is also a movement disorder and is far more dangerous and of paramount importance. Movement disorders presenting anew in the ED require an immediate neurologic assessment.[18,29,31,32] Many neurologists will first characterize the abnormal movement—hypokinetic or hyperkinetic—and ask themselves whether it may harm the patient. In several of these conditions, there is a perfect setup for the development of a critical (and even life-threatening) condition. Severe dystonia may cause aspiration, falling is possible with severe choreoathetosis, and freezing may cause profound rhabdomyolysis. New onset movement abnormalities—twitching, jerking, tremors, or spasms—will bring a patient into the ED. Many movement disorders are drug induced, but some point toward a clinical syndrome. As many physicians (and patients) know, medication effects are the most likely cause of tremors, but tremors are rarely severe enough to present the problem to an emergency physician.

When a patient with a florid movement disorder enters the ED, the following questions should be asked: What drug is the patient taking that could be implicated? What drug is the patient not taking that could cause these movements? What could these movements do to airway protection, respiration or circulatory stability? How much muscle breakdown is actually occurring and are protective measures in place? What intervention can be immediately successful? What metabolic derangements should be sought that can be caused by this movement disorder? These priorities are discussed in this chapter.

Principles

The first core principle is to diagnose the movement disorder. Some simple characteristics are shown in Figure 5.1. Not infrequently there are combinations of movement abnormalities, and a definitive opinion may have to wait. Neurologists may just

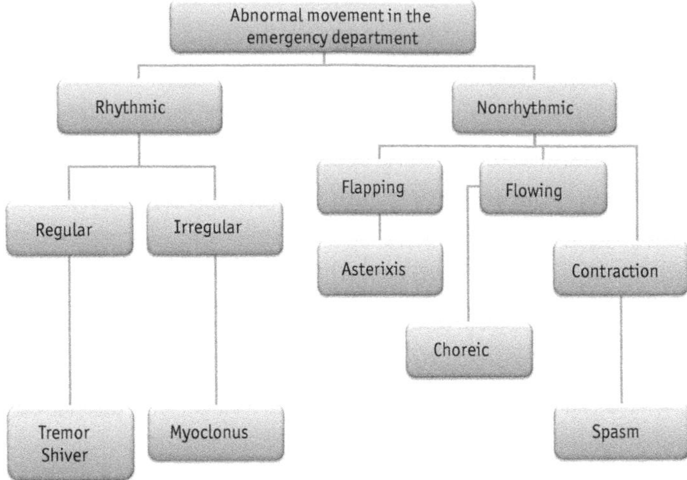

Figure 5.1 Simple characterization of acute movement disorder.

embarrassingly call it fidgets or some poorly defined pickiness or restlessness. Strange functional movement disorders are not that uncommon.

Generally, it is most practical to divide the movement disorder up into two main categories. Hypokinetic movement disorders are mostly Parkinson's disease or neurodegenerative disorders. Parkinsonism (as opposed to Parkinson's disease) refers to clinical features—often very prominently so—associated with other disorders. These are progressive supranuclear palsy, multiple system atrophy, Lewy body dementia, corticobasal degeneration, and the frontotemporal dementias. Clinical clues that can point away from typical Parkinson's disease are presence of cerebellar ataxia and orthostatic hypotension or other overt dysautonomic symptomatology. Obstructive airway disease causing stridor may play a role in advanced Parkinson's disease but is far more often seen in multisystem atrophy.

Occasionally, a patient with a known Parkinson's disease presenting in the ED may turn out to have progressive supranuclear palsy. These are patients with symptoms of "Parkinson's disease" who repeatedly visit the ED with falls. Often the history discloses a poor response to levodopa therapy. The diagnosis is clear when the patient is unable to track a finger vertically (particularly downward) but eyes move vertically with rapid head movements, proving the supranuclear nature of the clinical sign. There is very marked loss of facial mimicry and blinking. A marked atrophic brainstem on a regular CT scan may further point to this common mimicker of Parkinson's disease. Parkinsonism can also occur from drugs such as psychotropics and dopamine receptor antagonists.

The hyperkinetic disorders are usually part of a large variety of very unusual disorders, and their presentation requires some observation and deliberation to come to a diagnosis. The hyperkinetic disorders can present as chorea, ballism, athetosis, dystonia, tremor, and tics. Chorea is mostly a fluent purposeless movement, large in amplitude; and when it involves proximal muscles or abdomen and becomes more extreme, it is classified as ballism.[8,30] When it is unilateral (hemiballism) it is often acute and due to a stroke.[14] Dystonia is a sustained muscle cramplike movement.

The second core principle is that many tremors and jerks may be due to end-stage liver or kidney disease. These movements may be seen in patients with liver or kidney disease and who have variable attentiveness. Even in a drowsy patient, it is possible to find asterixis when arms are lifted with holding wrists and fingers in an extended position and it may be seen in the tongue and when puckering the lips—most typically however asterixis are brief, arrhythmic up and down flaps of hands and fingers. Stuporous patients may also demonstrate widespread (multifocal) myoclonic jerks. Myoclonus is a repetitive, irregular, quick jerk in several muscle groups, often moving the limb. It may be associated with action tremor (voluntary movement with increasing tremor amplitude reaching a target) or postural tremor (tremor at beginning and end of movement). These symptoms are very common, yet surprisingly, seldom recognized as such because they require certain positioning (asterixis) or close and prolonged observation (myoclonus). Patients with long-standing hypercapnia, or renal or liver disease, may likely have these movements, which will only disappear with improvement of liver, kidney, or lung function.

The third core principle is to determine the potential consequences of these movement disorders if they do not resolve quickly. Prolonged rigidity causes rhabdomyolysis and requires serial creatine phosphokinase (CPK) values. A single CPK may be elevated in the 100s and may seem right, but follow-up value may be in the 1000s or 10,000s.[16] Extremely high CPK values and dehydration (easily measured by abnormal blood urea nitrogen [BUN]/creatinine ratio) will lead to further worsening of creatinine values and may lead to acute renal injury and oliguria. Therefore, urine production (and inspection of color) needs attention in any patients with hypokinetic emergencies.

Another immediate concern is markedly reduced chest elastance, which leads to atelectasis and hypoxemia. As a general rule, restrictive pulmonary disease begins at a point where there is severe rigidity and marked bradykinesia. Pulmonary function studies have convincingly shown improvement, particularly of inspiratory flow, after levodopa administration. Conversely, acute respiratory failure may occur with withdrawal of dopamine agonists and may occur rapidly, with labored breathing, within 24 hours of stoppage. Aspiration in Parkinson's disease is very common and a direct result of delayed swallowing. Marked dysphagia, however, is not a feature of Parkinson's disease and is seen more typically in neurodegenerative diseases with parkinsonism. Failure to clear secretions with poor, inadequate swallowing leads to acute mucus plugging and profound aspiration that rapidly leads to pneumonia or acute respiratory distress syndrome.[36] These complications, not the neurologic manifestations, make these disorders critical. Finally, prolonged immobilization from protracted recovery can easily lead to decubital ulcers, deep venous thrombosis and pulmonary emboli. Good outcome, therefore, can only be achieved with full support and rapid reversal of the source of complications.

In Practice

Once a movement disorder is obvious, a number of considerations should come to mind (Figure 5.2). Several acute movement disorders should be considered that could point to a structural lesion and justify an MRI scan. Paroxysmal dyskinesias,

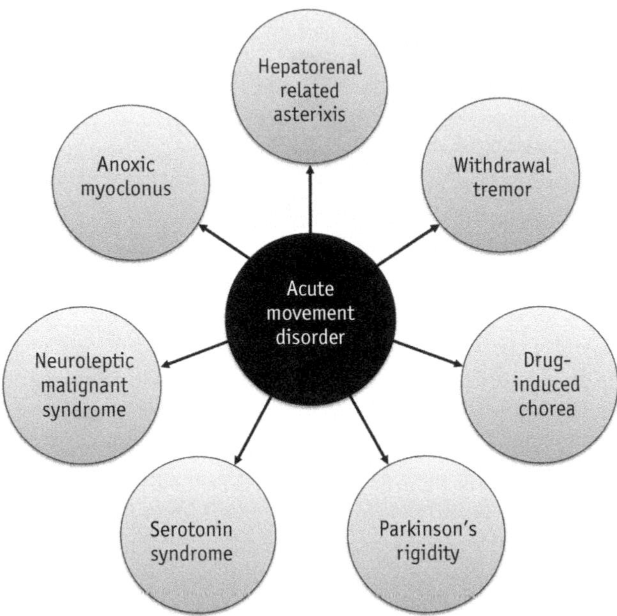

Figure 5.2 Common considerations in acute movement disorder.

whether dystonia, chorea, or athetosis, could be due to a secondary cause. Toxicity from overdose is a common occurrence. All drug-induced movement disorders are self-limiting, but there are quite a few. Parkinsonism can be caused by nearly all neuroleptics (clozapine and quetiapine are the only ones without these potential side effects). Parkinsonism has been described with high doses of antiemetics such as the dopamine-blocking drugs metoclopramide, prochlorperazine, and promethazine.

Several major disorders require full discussion here. They are rare, frequently unrecognized, recognized late, or—worse—known but insufficiently treated. Some generalizations in the available treatment options may apply here. Options are shown in Table 5.1. Treatment of the primary disorder is comparatively simple and again the appearance of a medical complication is what makes these disorders problematic.

Most patients with severe movement disorders are best helped with stopping the offending agent, and that may take time. This may be too long if the patient is under considerable distress, and escalating doses of benzodiazepines may help (usually lorazepam 2–4 mg IV). If the manifestations are severe and possibly injurious and causing marked sweating, tachycardia, and hypertension, it makes sense to temporarily intubate the patient and to sedate with a midazolam infusion titrating to a calm state. Akathisia may also be quite disabling when the patient moves virtually continuously. The first option is propranolol, clonidine, or amantadine and effect may be seen in 12–24 hours. Acute dystonia can be best treated with clonazepam (2–12 mg daily) or clozapine (200–400 mg daily). The combination of diphenhydramine 25 mg IV or benztropine (1–4 mg IV) is very effective initially, and some have argued to continue these anticholinergic agents for 2 weeks. A single dose of IV valium has been useful in

Table 5.1 **Treatment of Hyperkinetic Movement Disorders**

Movement Disorder	*Medication Class*	*Medication*	*Initial Daily Dose, mg*	*Recommended Maximum Daily Dose, mg*
Chorea	Neuroleptic	Haloperidol	0.5	8
		Risperidone	0.5	6
	Benzodiazepine	Clonazepam	0.5	6
Myoclonus	Antiepileptic	Valproic acid	750	Titrate to serum level
		Levetiracetam	500	3,000
		Primidone	12.5	750
	Benzodiazepine	Clonazepam	0.5	6
Tics	Neuroleptic	Haloperidol	0.5	8
		Risperidone	0.5	6
Dystonia	Anticholinergic	Benztropine mesylate	1	6
		Diphenhydramine	25	400

Source: Modified after Robottom, Factor and Weiner.[31]

children. Acute serotonin syndrome and neuroleptic malignant syndrome have specific treatments and are discussed below.

MYOCLONUS STATUS

Emergency physicians will likely see severe myoclonus commonly. This is because many patients with severe anoxic-ischemic encephalopathy may go through the ED. It is hard to miss, easy to treat, but often misjudged as convulsive status epilepticus. The muscle contractions are brief, of small amplitude, but can be forceful and shocklike and completely different from a tonic–clonic seizure even when seen in the resolving phase. The movements are usually chaotic and arrhythmic. Myoclonus is due to severe destruction in multiple cortical layers and due to continuous disinhibition. (Recall occasional myoclonic jerk with syncope, but here it is continuous and unrelenting.) Myoclonus is touch sensitive. It may also originate from the basal ganglia, brainstem, or spinal cord but when the insult is a severe anoxic-ischemic brain injury, all of these locations may be involved. Myoclonus status in a comatose patient is a strong indicator of poor prognosis. It should be differentiated from isolated myoclonic jerk, other types of seizures, and an action myoclonus of Lance–Adams. Lance–Adams syndrome frequently follows respiratory arrest and becomes evident after awakening or is present in a patient who has never been comatose after cardiopulmonary resuscitation.

Drug-induced myoclonus may involve manifestations of first exposure or appear after toxic doses. Drugs that can put a patient into myoclonus status are the selective serotonin reuptake inhibitors (SSRIs) and lithium. There should be specific inquiry for use of lithium and perhaps even a lithium level to exclude this possibility. Patients with lithium become agitated, with development of fasciculations and cerebellar dysfunction, and may have initially choreiform movements as part of the clinical manifestation. This is rapidly followed by seizures and coma when the serum levels reach 3.5 mEq/L (a three-fold increase above the normal target range). Myoclonus is an underrecognized manifestation of lithium intoxication, which may induce ocular myoclonus in all directions and axial myoclonus. Generalized myoclonus is common in acute metabolic derangements, but more usually at end-stage organ failure such as hepatic and renal disease. It has been observed in hypernatremia, hypomagnesemia, and nonketotic hyperglycemia. Unusual causes are heat stroke, decompression injury, and pesticide exposure. The toxic exposure may have caused permanent damage to the cortex and basal ganglia.

ACUTE DYSTONIC REACTION

The word "dystonia" is reserved for movements characterized by a persistent posture in one extremity. There is sustained patterned spasm but normal tone in between. The positions may be bizarre and can be in both limbs and trunk. In the ED, it is useful to distinguish between a generalized or focal dystonia and whether dystonia occurs at rest. A form of dystonia is ocular deviation (oculogyric crisis). Oculogyric crisis may be associated with backward or lateral flexion of the neck, and the tongue may protrude. The deviation of the eyes upward, sideways, or downward is held for several minutes and can only for a brief moment be corrected by effort. This eye movement is commonly drug induced, and discontinuation of the drug is rapidly successful. Oculogyric crisis do occur in serious neurologic conditions such as bilateral paramedian thalamic infarction, multiple sclerosis, head injury, and tumors in the ventricles. Drugs causing oculogyric crisis and oromandibular dyskinesis include phenothiazines and many of the antipsychotic drugs, but also carbamazepine, gabapentin, lithium, ondansetron, and perhaps best known, metoclopramide. Any physician seeing patients with acute dystonia should consider Wilson's disease, particularly when patients are 20–30 years old. Additional findings are artificial grin (retracted lips) and brown iris in previously blue-eyed persons. Diagnostic tests include reduced serum ceruloplasmin level (in 5% of patients it is normal), Kayser-Fleischer rings under slit lamp, and increased signal in basal ganglia and cortex on MRI.

Acute dystonic reactions are often successfully treated with IV or oral administration of anticholinergics (benztropine) or antihistaminic agents (diphenhydramine). In the most severe cases, treatment may include IV infusion of clonidine or midazolam.[7,22,25] Other laboratory tests may be abnormal and include acidosis, hyperkalemia, hypocalcemia, and BUN.[20]

STATUS DYSTONICUS

This disorder is recognized clinically as a sustained contraction of multiple muscle groups and may cause repetitive twisting movements or unusual postures. It may lead to exhaustion and pain from muscle damage or joint overstretching. When it involves shoulder, face, or oropharyngeal muscles, it becomes a neuromedical critical illness. Trismus can be very severe, dislocating the jaw, and often there is lateral flexion or extreme retrocollis. The patient is in distress, and the extreme grimacing is often misinterpreted as pain—but there is none.[2]

The condition may occur de novo (e.g., drug reaction) or worsening in patients with known focal dystonias (e.g., infection, sudden drug effect withdrawal). Haloperidol and also dopamine receptor blockers, clozapine, intrathecal baclofen pump failure are all known triggers.

The first line of action is intubation and sedation, particularly if the patient demonstrates pharyngeal, laryngeal, and diaphragmatic dystonia.[2,3,5,21,34] The next step is fluid resuscitation with multiple boluses of crystalloids and temperature control with cooling blankets or cooling pads. Neuromuscular-blocking agents may be used initially for 24–48 hours. The dystonic contractions are best treated with oral or IV clonidine (3–5 mg/kg) administered every 3 hours and may be supplemented with IV midazolam or IV lorazepam. Initial CPK levels may be dramatic and high (10,000's). The CPK levels are the best monitoring laboratory tests, and resolution is quick after treatment. Gabapentin and baclofen in oral doses have been concomitantly administered.[15] Antiepileptic drugs have not been useful, even in combinations. Deep brain stimulation is a last-resort option and cases are on record with successful management.[17,20]

NEUROLEPTIC MALIGNANT SYNDROME

Neuroleptics, metoclopramide, droperidol, and promethazine cause this syndrome, most similar to parkinsonism. Incidence rates for neuroleptic malignant syndrome range from 0.02% to 3% among patients taking these agents, and thus it is not entirely negligible. Neuroleptic malignant syndrome is most often seen with high-potency neuroleptic agents (e.g., haloperidol, fluphenazine), but may occur with the atypical antipsychotic drugs (e.g., clozapine, risperidone, olanzapine) and antiemetic drugs (e.g., metoclopramide, promethazine). An initially high dose, recent major dose increase, and a reaction to the first dose are common triggers. Concomitant use of lithium may increase the risk. Fever, rigidity, and rhabdomyolysis and dysautonomic signs such as tachycardia, tachypnea, and profuse sweating are key findings identical to parkinsonism-hyperpyrexia syndrome, which is a result of sudden withdrawal of Parkinson's drugs. Patients have been described as warm and stiff. Fever and dehydration will lead to other laboratory abnormalities including hypocalcemia, hypomagnesemia, and hypernatremia. Serum creatinine may rise quickly if rhabdomyolysis—again CPK is important—is not treated with high fluid intake. Treatment is dantrolene 1 mg/kg IV and repeat to maximal dose of 10 mg/kg, followed by an oral dose of 4 mg/kg daily for 7 days. (Note that there is a tendency to wean the drug too early when patient and CPK have markedly improved.) Administration of sodium bicarbonate should be guided by arterial blood gas analysis. Cooling the patient is an essential part of treatment, and use of cooling devices is very effective.

SEROTONIN SYNDROME

Serotonin syndrome is a rapidly increasing disorder but remain poorly recognized. The SSRIs currently in use that can induce this syndrome are sertraline, fluoxetine, fluvoxamine, paroxetine, and citalopram.[3] Serotonin syndrome does not occur (or only rarely) with ingestion of bupropion. Bupropion is another commonly used antidepressant and is also used for smoking cessation. It selectively inhibits neuronal reuptake of dopamine and norepinephrine and may have indirect effects on serotonergic receptors. The drug in high dose will cause tachycardia, slurred speech, dry skin, ataxia, and seizures, but no hyperreflexia or hyperthermia following overdose. The serotonergic effects of bupropion have been debated.

A serotonin syndrome may present within days of administration of a serotonin reuptake inhibitor and not infrequently as a result of coingestion of a drug that reduces its clearance or as a result of a suicide attempt. Mortality can be substantial because the condition can lead to metabolic acidosis, rhabdomyolysis, acute liver failure, renal failure, and—in the most extreme cases—disseminated intravascular coagulation. Serotonin syndrome seldom is in the differential diagnosis in an elderly patient because acute agitation is often attributed to preexisting dementia. The patient will not improve if the drug is not discontinued. Patients are often hyperactive with myoclonus (predominant legs), markedly rigid with hyperreflexia, and may be febrile and with a leucocytosis. Several drugs have been implicated (Table 5.2). Fentanyl (or any opioid) is an underrecognized trigger in this syndrome, and some patients on this drug even have been treated accidentally with opioids, worsening the syndrome. Cyproheptadine (32 mg daily in 3–6 divided doses) is used mostly in patients with severe dysautonomia. Some experts have suggested an initial dose of 20 mg cyproheptadine followed by 2 mg every 2 hours. Additional intramuscular administration of 100 mg of chlorpromazine is often considered. Most of the management will be focused on control of the autonomic

Table 5.2 **Drugs Reported to Cause Serotonin Syndrome**

Drug
Monoamine oxidase inhibitors
Selective serotonin reuptake inhibitors
Serotonin-norepinephrine reuptake inhibitors
Tricyclic antidepressants
L-tryptophan
Buspirone hydrochloride
Fentanyl
3, 4-Methylenedioxymethamphetamine (ecstasy)
Lysergic acid diethylamide
Amphetamines
Cocaine

Source: Modified from Robottom, Weiner and Factor.[31]

instability, and patients may have fluctuating blood pressures. Liberal use of fluids is essential to avoid rapid dehydration and to reduce the effect of rhabdomyolysis on the kidney. Severe rigidity can also cause poor movement of the chest wall, compromising ventilation. If there is severe rigidity, benzodiazepines are the drugs of choice. Propranolol, bromocriptine, and dantrolene are not recommended. The prognosis of serotonin syndrome is usually very good.

ADVANCED PARKINSON'S AND NEURODEGENERATIVE DISEASES

A considerable proportion of patients with advanced Parkinson's disease will frequent the ED. Some will have sustained a fall, and dyskinesias may be obvious. In many of these patients, motor fluctuations have been a major problem after prolonged use of levodopa and carbidopa. Some of it is a peak-dose levodopa effect. Modification of the dose is needed and some strategies are shown in Table 5.3. At times, patients present emergently in a delirium with hallucinations and delusions. Hallucination often involves persons in the room and may be associated with paranoia. It may become too severe to handle at home, with family members bringing the patient to the ED for management. Usually, Parkinson's drugs can be identified as the main culprit. Most movement disorder experts recommend: (1) simplifying the drug regimen and eliminating drugs of uncertain indication, (2) halving the dose of dopamine agonists, and (3) administering quetiapine starting at a low dose (25 mg) gradually and increasing the dose up to 200 mg at night. Admission may be needed to protect the patient from doing harm. Some of these recommendations can be started, but the patient would need to be seen by a movement disorder expert. As alluded to earlier, patients may present with "Parkinson's disease" but more detailed examination will reveal marked cerebellar dysfunction with gait and limb ataxia, supranuclear gaze palsy, slowing of oculomotor saccades, and difficulty initiating saccades as part of multiple system atrophy. The dysautonomia and cerebellar ataxia may have caused repeated syncopes or frequent falls.

Table 5.3 **Strategies to Treat Motor Fluctuations**

End-of-dose deterioration	(1) Increase LD/CD (2) Substitute sustained-release LD/CD (3) Add dopamine agonist (4) Add COMT inhibitor
"Off" dystonia (Nighttime)	(1) Add sustained-release LD/CD at bedtime (2) Add dopamine agonist at bedtime
Peak-dose dyskinesia	(1) Smaller doses of levodopa taken more frequently (2) Add dopamine agonist, decrease levodopa (3) Add amantadine

LD/CD = levodopa/carbidopa; COMT = catechol-*O*-methyltransferase.

Source: Adapted from Ahlskog.[1]

ACUTE PARKINSONIAN EMERGENCIES

The causes of acute parkinsonism are shown in Table 5.4. Very few neurologists have seen these etiologies and many of these associations are unconfirmed. Cases are on record with rapidly worsening parkinsonism and acute hydrocephalus. Akinesia may improve with shunting, but not in all patients.[31] Acute freezing of gait has also been reported, with acute strokes in expected areas such as the substantia nigra, but these are exceptional circumstances. The main manifestations are acute akinesia or acute dyskinesia. Acute akinesia is associated with hyperthermia and is also known

Table 5.4 **Causes of Acute Parkinsonism**

Cause
Structural
Stroke
Subdural hematoma
Hydrocephalus
Drug induced
Neuroleptics
Antiepileptics
Antidepressants
Chemotherapeutic agents
Amiodarone
Toxic
1-Methyl-1-4-phenyl-4-proprionoxypiperidine
Carbon monoxide
Carbon disulfide
Manganese
Cyanide
Methanol
Infectious
Viral encephalitis
Human immunodeficiency virus
Whipple disease
Postinfectious
Metabolic
Central pontine myelinolysis
Hereditary
Wilson's disease
Rapid-onset dystonia-parkinsonism
Psychiatric
Catatonia
Psychogenic

Source: From Robottom, Weiner and Factor.[31]

Table 5.5 **Management of Symptoms in Acute Parkinson's Syndrome**

Orthostatic hypotension	Crystalloids (500–1000 ml IV) Florinef (0.4 mg orally) Midodrine (10–40 mg daily) Pyridostigmine (60–240 mg daily)
Gastroparesis	Metoclopramide (5–20 mg) Pyridostigmine (30–60 mg) Erythromycin (250 mg q.i.d.)

Source: Data from Benarroch.[4]

as parkinsonism-hyperpyrexia syndrome or akinetic crisis.[12,23,26,27] Acute parkinsonism has also been described with acute toxins (organophosphates, sarin, cyanide, and methanol). Most causes are related to sudden withdrawal of medication, a recent surgery, or—for some unexplained reason in elderly patients — undergoing orthopedic surgery. The syndrome does also occur in patients with olivopontocerebellar atrophy. Clinical features are increased core temperature that may reach hyperthermia values (40°C), marked rigidity, and dysautonomia.[4,25] The dysautonomia is usually not initially appreciated but may evolve into a clinical picture with tachycardia, anhidrosis or sweating, dysperistalsis of the gut or even adynamic ileus, and marked blood pressure changes, all associated with rhabdomyolysis as a result of constantly contracting skeletal muscles.[11] Rhabdomyolysis may lead to diffuse intravascular coagulation. The only way that levodopa withdrawal syndrome, neuroleptic malignant syndrome, and malignant hyperthermia distinguish themselves is by a known underlying disease (i.e., respectively known Parkinson's disease, known schizophrenia, or a known myopathy). Specific treatment includes levodopa, bromocriptine, and dantrolene. Many patients respond well to dantrolene. The general management of acute autonomic failure is shown in Table 5.5.

ACUTE TORTICOLLIS

A nontraumatic subluxation of the atlantoaxial joint due to inflammation from a spreading infection may cause acute torticollis (also known as Grisel's syndrome).[10,33,35] It is common in children, but may occur in adults; and neurologists are not often familiar with this syndrome. On examination, the chin is down and to one side. A CT scan will show a significant C1-C2 rotary subluxation. Treatment is antibiotics (it often occurs after tonsillectomy for tonsillitis) and muscle relaxants. Cervical spinal tumors and posterior fossa tumors have been associated with torticollis.[19]

FUNCTIONAL MOVEMENT DISORDERS

The diagnosis of functional (psychogenic) movement disorders has no place in the ED, so patients may need to be seen in a clinic or briefly observed and videotaped in a hospital setting. Careful examination and consultation with colleagues may be needed

Table 5.6 **Clinical Clues Suggesting a Functional Movement Disorder**

Inconsistency
Increase with attention, decrease with distraction
Entrainment of tremor to the frequency of repetitive movements
Variability of phenomenology during examination
Selective disability or functional disability out of proportion to examination findings
Incongruency
Mixed movement disorders
Atypical stimulus sensitivity
Paroxysmal attacks
False weakness
False sensory signs
Deliberate slowness
Suggestibility

Source: Adapted from Gupta and Lang.[13]

to diagnose these abnormalities with certainty.[6,9,28] Clues are movement disorders that disappear when the patient is not directly observed and it can be proven with surveillance video monitoring, or that the movement disorder disappears with "lying on the hands." Some criteria are shown in Table 5.6.[24]

TRIAGE

Most movement disorder emergencies may need close observation in an ICU. This will provide adequate attention to vital signs, hydration, and protection of airway patency and pulmonary function. Any of these major emergencies may rapidly develop a pulmonary infection that may result in sepsis. Frequently, patients with severe Parkinson's disease have urinary retention or a urinary tract infection that may progress to a full urosepsis. Many patients in this condition may have poor bowel movement and are prone to adynamic ileus. Management on a regular ward is just too complex for many of these patients and often close participation of a neurologist, a movement disorder expert, or a neurointensivist is needed to provide the best solutions and evaluation for a cause, if not yet known.

Putting It All Together

- Most movement disorders in the ED are hypokinetic.
- Most movement disorders of importance are drug related.
- Movement disorders may indicate major organ failure.
- Malignant neuroleptic syndrome and serotonin syndrome are acute movement disorders with specific treatment.

- Management of advanced Parkinson's disease is a common consult, but may require admission.
- Many deteriorating patients with Parkinson's disease may have a lingering infection.
- Withdrawal of levodopa in established Parkinson's disease may lead to a life-threatening illness with hyperthermia and rigidity and all its medical consequences.

By the Way

- Acute dystonias are often drug related.
- Most movement disorders remain unexplained.
- Acute brain injury is an uncommon cause of movement disorders.
- Benzodiazepines may help in many poorly defined movement disorders.
- Severe movement disorders may need aggressive sedation and intubation.

Acute Movement Disorders by the Numbers

- ~90% of myoclonus status is due to anoxic-ischemic brain injury.
- ~80% of acute hemiballism is due to ischemic stroke.
- ~70% will develop dyskinesias after 5 years of levodopa treatment.
- ~50% of patients with dopamine-blocking agents develop tardive dyskinesias.
- ~50% of patients with essential tremor remember a family history.
- ~30% of patients with multiple system atrophy respond to levodopa.

References

1. Ahlskog JE. *The Parkinson's Disease Treatment Book: Partnering with Your Doctor to Get the Most from Your Medications.* New York: Oxford University Press; 2005.
2. Allen NM, Lin JP, Lynch T, King MD. Status dystonicus: a practice guide. *Dev Med Child Neurol* 2014;56:105–112.
3. Angelini L, Nardocci N, Estienne M, et al. Life-threatening dystonia-dyskinesias in a child: successful treatment with bilateral pallidal stimulation. *Mov Disord* 2000;15: 1010–1012.
4. Benarroch EE. The clinical approach to autonomic failure in neurological disorders. *Nat Rev Neurol* 2014;10:396–407.
5. Campbell D. The management of acute dystonic reactions. *Australian Prescriber* 2001;24:19–20.
6. Dallocchio C, Marangi A, Tinazzi M. Functional or psychogenic movement disorders: an endless enigmatic tale. *Front Neurol.* 2015;6:37.
7. Dalvi A, Fahn S, Ford B. Intrathecal baclofen in the treatment of dystonic storm. *Mov Disord* 1998;13:611–612.
8. Dewey RB, Jr., Jankovic J. Hemiballism-hemichorea: clinical and pharmacologic findings in 21 patients. *Arch Neurol* 1989;46:862–867.
9. Fahn S, Olanow CW. "Psychogenic movement disorders": they are what they are. *Mov Disord* 2014;29:853–856.

10. Gourin CG, Kaper B, Abdu WA, Donegan JO. Nontraumatic atlanto-axial subluxation after retropharyngeal cellulitis: Grisel's syndrome. *Am J Otolaryngol* 2002;23:60–65.
11. Granner MA, Wooten GF. Neuroleptic malignant syndrome or parkinsonism hyperpyrexia syndrome. *Semin Neurol* 1991;11:228–235.
12. Guneysel O, Onultan O, Onur O. Parkinson's disease and the frequent reasons for emergency admission. *Neuropsychiatr Dis Treat* 2008;4:711–714.
13. Gupta A, Lang AE. Psychogenic movement disorders. *Curr Opin Neurol* 2009;22:430–436.
14. Handley A, Medcalf P, Hellier K, Dutta D. Movement disorders after stroke. *Age Ageing* 2009;38:260–266.
15. Jankovic J, Penn AS. Severe dystonia and myoglobinuria. *Neurology* 1982;32:1195–1197.
16. Jankovic J. Treatment of hyperkinetic movement disorders. *Lancet Neurol* 2009;8:844–856.
17. Jech R, Bares M, Urgosik D, et al. Deep brain stimulation in acute management of status dystonicus. *Mov Disord* 2009;24:2291–2292.
18. Kipps CM, Fung VS, Grattan-Smith P, de Moore GM, Morris JG. Movement disorder emergencies. *Mov Disord* 2005;20:322–334.
19. Kumandas S, Per H, Gumus H, et al. Torticollis secondary to posterior fossa and cervical spinal cord tumors: report of five cases and literature review. *Neurosurg Rev* 2006;29:333–338; discussion 338.
20. Lumsden DE, Lundy C, Fairhurst C, Lin JP. Dystonia Severity Action Plan: a simple grading system for medical severity of status dystonicus and life-threatening dystonia. *Dev Med Child Neurol* 2013;55:671–672.
21. Manji H, Howard RS, Miller DH, et al. Status dystonicus: the syndrome and its management. *Brain* 1998;121(Pt 2):243–252.
22. Mariotti P, Fasano A, Contarino MF, et al. Management of status dystonicus: our experience and review of the literature. *Mov Disord* 2007;22:963–968.
23. Mizuno Y, Takubo H, Mizuta E, Kuno S. Malignant syndrome in Parkinson's disease: concept and review of the literature. *Parkinsonism Relat Disord* 2003;9 Suppl 1:S3–9.
24. Morgante F, Edwards MJ, Espay AJ. Psychogenic movement disorders. *Continuum (Minneap Minn)* 2013;19:1383–1396.
25. Narayan RK, Loubser PG, Jankovic J, Donovan WH, Bontke CF. Intrathecal baclofen for intractable axial dystonia. *Neurology* 1991;41:1141–1142.
26. Onofrj M, Bonanni L, Cossu G, et al. Emergencies in parkinsonism: akinetic crisis, life-threatening dyskinesias, and polyneuropathy during L-Dopa gel treatment. *Parkinsonism Relat Disord* 2009;15 Suppl 3:S233–236.
27. Onofrj M, Thomas A. Acute akinesia in Parkinson disease. *Neurology* 2005;64:1162–1169.
28. Peckham EL, Hallett M. Psychogenic movement disorders. *Neurol Clin* 2009;27:801–819, vii.
29. Poston KL, Frucht SJ. Movement disorder emergencies. *J Neurol* 2008;255 Suppl 4:2–13.
30. Ristic A, Marinkovic J, Dragasevic N, Stanisavljevic D, Kostic V. Long-term prognosis of vascular hemiballismus. *Stroke* 2002;33:2109–2111.
31. Robottom BJ, Weiner WJ, Factor SA. Movement disorders emergencies. Part 1: hypokinetic disorders. *Arch Neurol* 2011;68:567–572.
32. Robottom BJ, Factor SA, Weiner WJ. Movement disorders emergencies. Part 2: hyperkinetic disorders. *Arch Neurol* 2011;68:719–724.
33. Samuel D, Thomas DM, Tierney PA, Patel KS. Atlanto-axial subluxation (Grisel's syndrome) following otolaryngological diseases and procedures. *J Laryngol Otol* 1995;109:1005–1009.
34. Weiner WJ, Goetz CG, Nausieda PA, Klawans HL. Respiratory dyskinesias: extrapyramidal dysfunction and dyspnea. *Ann Intern Med* 1978;88:327–331.
35. Welinder NR, Hoffmann P, Hakansson S. Pathogenesis of non-traumatic atlanto-axial subluxation (Grisel's syndrome). *Eur Arch Otorhinolaryngol* 1997;254:251–254.
36. Woodford H, Walker R. Emergency hospital admissions in idiopathic Parkinson's disease. *Mov Disord* 2005;20:1104–1108.

6

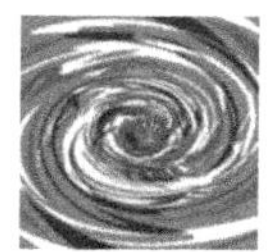

Triaging Seizures and Spells

In the ED, a seizure is what it is—a seizure. Patients may enter the critical pod after a seizure has been observed outside the hospital or may be in a postictal state or on the verge of a second seizure. The emergency physician is usually the first to intervene. The neurologist is often the one who evaluates the patient after initial management. In the ED, a large category of patients with seizures are infants with febrile seizures and some have otitis media as a co-diagnosis. A second common group seen in the ED are middle-aged adults.[19] In this group, drugs and alcohol plays a role. And furthermore, patients with epilepsy are frequently in the ED, often as a result of poor medication compliance.[2,18]

Descriptions from bystanders may be helpful but are seldom detailed enough to tell the full story. Therefore, there are other clinical findings or even laboratory characteristics that could point toward the nature of the seizure. In any event, if there is a high likelihood of a generalized tonic–clonic seizure, an aggressive diagnostic approach is warranted.[23] There are many questions that are immediately apparent: How do we recognize different types of seizures? When is intubation necessary? What are the complications of aggressive management? What is the practical use of EEG monitoring and how is it of value? How do we avoid misdiagnosis of epilepsy?[26]

This chapter provides a template for emergency room physicians and also neurologists called to see a patient with a presumed seizure or some atypical spell or a possibly equally common pseudoepileptic seizure. Encountering "a strange spell" will beg the question "It is a seizure, stroke, syncope, or something else"? The fact remains there are many types of spells, and so many remain unexplained. Several patients may start with a seemingly innocuous spell that could be a seizure but then worsen and progress to a series of seizures. The current management of this neurocritical illness progressing to status epilepticus can be found in another volume (*Handling Difficult Situations*).

Principles

One of the first core principles is to consider the major categories of spells presenting in the ED. Many first responders and the admitting emergency physician may be convinced a seizure has occurred, but there may be healthy doubt with the consulted neurologist. When a diagnostic uncertainty remains, other causes need consideration and there are a few important ones.[25] This spectrum of spells is shown in Table 6.1 and Figure 6.1. For each spell, history should include questions about precipitating factors, a witnessed facial flush or pallor, feeling of irregular heart rate or "racing" and need to diurese, observed breathing pattern by bystanders (labored, apnea), and if there was an opportunity to get seriously hurt (fractures from fall). The examination should concentrate on changes in heart rate and blood pressure with position change. Further studies may include 24-hour urinary excretion of metanephrines, 5-hydroxyindoleacetic acid, and CT of the abdomen to look for pheochromocytoma or a PET scan for other neuroendocrine tumors. A spell might be a stroke albeit unusual. Some ischemic strokes involving the frontal and nondominant temporal lobe can produce new confusional behavior and memory lapses. A drug screen is imperative in most circumstances because spells may occur with illicit drug and alcohol use that is denied sometimes even by the accompanying family.

Table 6.1 **The Spectrum of Spells**

Type	*Clues*
Psychogenic	• Prior anxiety or depression • Increasing frequency (aggravation) • Strange and atypical
Endocrine tumor	• Pallor (pheochromocytoma) • Flushing (carcinoid) • Hypertension (pheochromocytoma) • Hypotension (carcinoid) • Hypoglycemia (insulinoma)
Seizures	• Staring (temporal lobe) • Automatisms (absences/nonconvulsive)
Stroke	• Unusual behavior (frontal lesion) • Memory lapse (nondominant temporal lobe lesion)
Syncope	• Pallor • Orthostatic hypotension • Cardiac arrhythmias • Dysautonomia • Baroreflex dysfunction
Drugs	• Illegal drug ingestion • Withdrawal of adrenergic inhibitor
Sudden falls	• History of narcolepsy • Drop attacks • Sudden loss of tone (atonic seizure)

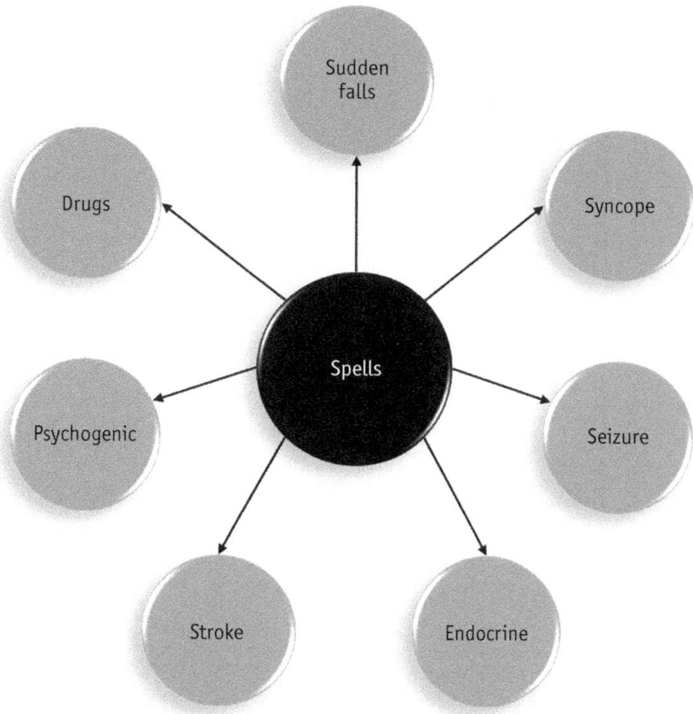

Figure 6.1 Common considerations in evaluation of spells.

Many patients have a syncope, and most physicians in the ED will assume a single syncopal episode can be attributed to neurally mediated syncope, such as a vasovagal attack, situational syncope, or carotid sinus syncope. In less than 1 of 10 patients, syncope is symptomatic of neurologic disease (see Chapter 3). Sometimes situations are far more complex than they seem. I recall a patient who had a vaguely described "spell" and was taken to the ED; he was found to be in marked hypercapnic respiratory failure and was intubated for laryngospasm with aspiration. I recall a patient seen on the cardiology ward and prepared for cardiac pacing when a major tongue bite was found.

Frequently, the clinical exercise is to put up a "pro and con" list when comparing seizures with syncope. Seizures often last much longer and rarely less than 30 seconds (syncopes are brief), auras may occur that may involve *déjà vu* and *jamais vu*, gustatory or olfactory hallucinations, and other feelings of sense of doom (syncope is the world closing in, darkening of vision, and muting sounds), stereotypic behavior may occur (a patient with syncope just falls to the ground), postictal confusion occurs for several minutes to an hour (recovery of alertness and composure is quick after a syncope), tongue bite and incontinence are common, and injuries to other parts of the body are frequent (rare with syncope). Perhaps the most distinguishing feature is a cry at seizure onset that sounds very ominous and the marked snoring or labored and loud breathing at resolution of the spell, none of which occurs with a syncope. Physicians should, however, be aware that both conditions can coexist in the rare occurrence of ictal bradycardia. Ictal bradycardia can cause significant hypotension and is sometimes seen with temporal lobe seizures. This condition can only be found with complex prolonged monitoring, and in fact some of these patients may need cardiac pacing.

The second core principle is to identify the cause of the seizure. Cause may not be obvious—but it is more important to first carefully consider whether there are potentially precipitating factors. Experts usually divide the causes into nonspecific predisposing factors, specific epileptogenic disturbances, and precipitating factors.[5]

Seizures may seem unifactorial, but it is more likely they are multifactorial. Many patients are susceptible to seizures and some changed circumstance pushes them through the threshold. Some patients are genetically predisposed, and it is known that seizures more often occur in first-degree relatives of patients with established epilepsy. A certain drug, a certain metabolic derangement, a certain stressful circumstance may incite cortical excitability and may then result in a clinical seizure in a predisposed patient. Hippocampal sclerosis is a common cause for (medically refractory) focal seizures. There are several acquired causes of seizures, but it is highly variable (10% in stroke, 70% in brain tumors, 20% in CNS infections—except in neurocysticercosis, where it reaches nearly 100%). Some situations that are comparatively common are listed in Table 6.2. One can anticipate that most seizures in the ED are seen in patients with known seizures. Many for some reason have changed medication dose, arbitrarily stopped medication, or had no access to medication. In some patients, a new-onset seizure is the first presentation of a cavernous angioma or arachnoid cyst. Glioma is notorious for presenting with a generalized tonic–clonic seizure but not vice versa. Some seizures are a result of taking an epileptogenic drug; the most well known are antibiotics (meropenem), antipsychotics, and antidepressants and often when high doses are prescribed.

Table 6.2 **Conditions That Predispose a Patient to Have a Seizure**

- Change in medication or discontinuation of medication in prior epileptic
- Acute or chronic subdural hematoma
- Glioma or metastasis
- New immunosuppression in transplant patient
- Hypertensive emergency and posterior reversible encephalopathy syndrome
- New-onset herpes simplex encephalitis
- Severe hyponatremia
- Severe hyperglycemia or hypoglycemia
- Environmental toxin
- Alcohol withdrawal
- Street drug

When a seizure is suspected, it is useful for the emergency physician to know what the neurologist knows. Here are some facts. A single seizure may not need immediate treatment. A well-known principle is that only two seizures do require immediate antiepileptic treatment. However, though it is also widely believed that a single seizure is not particularly harmful to the patient, this is a myth. A first time seizure can cause significant TBI and polytrauma. Unilateral or bilateral shoulder dislocations requiring surgery are well known. Seizures can cause potential harm due to systemic manifestations. A generalized tonic–clonic seizure may cause major dysautonomic features that may include tachycardia and hypertensive surge. This may cause, in a susceptible patient, demand ischemia evidenced by EKG changes and, in other patients, immediate development of laboratory abnormalities. What is usually underappreciated is that a generalized tonic–clonic seizure often produces an impressive mixed respiratory and metabolic acidosis, and serum pH can be below 7 if drawn minutes after the ictal phase has resolved. The metabolic component of the acidosis is usually caused by increased lactate and may also be associated with rhabdomyolysis. The respiratory component is entirely a result of upper airway obstruction and marked abnormality of respiratory drive (often prolonged apnea). Failure to recognize a severe acidosis and rhabdomyolysis may lead to cardiac arrhythmias and rapidly developing renal failure. Moreover, the anoxic episode during a generalized tonic–clonic seizure may result in secondary brain injury. Hypoxemia can be caused by aspiration or by upper airway obstruction associated with seizure itself. Both conditions can worsen a respiratory acidosis and be an additional component to the generalized acidosis.

The third core principle is that some patients may have to be intubated after a single seizure. Generally, most neurologists feel that patient with a generalized tonic–clonic seizure are unnecessarily intubated. This is a complicated issue with good arguments for both sides. Against rapid action is that the use of rapid-sequence intubation will paralyze the patient and make any visualization of seizures impossible. It is therefore theoretically possible that a patient who is in convulsive status epilepticus might be paralyzed and has ongoing seizures which can only be detected by an EEG. Arguments for rapid intubation are that patients may pool secretions rapidly, may aspirate, and are unable to protect their airway after a generalized tonic–clonic seizure. The respiratory distress after a generalized tonic–clonic seizure is not commonly appreciated. During the tonic phase, there is complete apnea with occasional escaping sounds until the clonic phase sets in. Then there are mostly brief inspiratory gasps until the patient enters a postictal phase in which there is loud, stertorous breathing that is associated with significant tracheal secretions. Nursing staff often recognize the large amount of tracheal secretions which is likely as a result of dysautonomic hypersecretion and may lead to aspiration. In some patients, there might even be vomiting after a generalized tonic–clonic seizure. This usually resolves within several minutes and can be best supported by moving the patient into a side position, with frequent suctioning to avoid further desaturation. There is no need to intubate the patient emergently, only if prompted by persistent oxygen desaturation on the pulse oximeter.

The fourth core principle is to immediately treat the patient with ongoing seizures, starting with IV loading of fosphenytoin and to place two large-bore IV catheters. Most of the time, a patient is treated with 20 mg/kg of phenytoin or fosphenytoin—whatever is available—and this is provided to most patients in a 30-minute infusion. These drugs do have a tendency to cause hypotension, but there are rarely cardiac arrhythmias of any concern. Brief discontinuation of the infusion and additional fluid bolus or a single IV dose of 200 mcg norepinephrine will correct the treatment associated hypotension. There is no immediate need in a patient who is in a postictal state to administer lorazepam; but if there has been a second seizure, 4 mg of lorazepam is likely to prevent further seizures. In general, the combination of lorazepam and fosphenytoin will avoid further seizures in the majority of patients with recurrent seizures or early status epilepticus.

The fifth core principle is to recognize that patients with pseudoseizures can be easily overtreated. Nearly, 50% have previously visited EDs or have been previously admitted.[17] There are multiple examples of patients who have been diagnosed with recurrent seizures not responding to medication, not responding to IV drugs, who were intubated and developed iatrogenic complications from line placement, overuse of antiepileptic drugs, and rapidly developing hypotension. Fatality associated with treatment of psychogenic nonepileptic seizures has been reported and is understandable if recurrent seizures are aggressively managed.

The clinical recognition of a pseudoseizure involves three aspects. There are differences between the preictal phase, the ictal phase, and the postictal phase (Table 6.3). In general, in fake seizures, patients have their eyes closed, the seizure is of long duration, is asynchronous with alternately stopping and starting of the flapping movement, and often the head turns to left and right. Patient can have rapid breathing, but none of it is stertorous as in a generalized tonic–clonic seizure, and usually during the seizure rather than in a postictal phase as in a real seizure. In these patients, arterial blood gas, CPK, and prolactin will all be normal. A tongue bite can be found, and there also might be incontinence. The tongue bite is usually the tip of the tongue rather than the lateral portion of the tongue.

The sixth core principle is that the availability of EEG in the ED with EEG data sent to a skilled neurologist would be an ideal situation in the following circumstances: (1) detection of nonconvulsive status epilepticus in unexplained unresponsiveness. The yield remains very low if examination does not show any clinical hints such as nystagmoid eyemovements, eyelid twitching, or jaw or mouth twitching, (2) identification of nonconvulsive status versus postictal stupor, (3) recognition of absent correlation of movements with simultaneous EEG recordings.[1,7,11,21,22]

Nearly, 60% of children could be discharged from the ED using EEG.[6] Studies looking at abbreviated EEG montages have generally been disappointing. Often times, these urgent EEGs with abbreviated montages will show indeterminate, nonspecific patterns, and for many neurologists, it is difficult to be definitive without the full array of recording. Neurologist and emergency physicians will both likely cavil over its

Table 6.3 **Differentiating Real from Fake Seizures**

	Real	***Fake***
Preictus	Usually no triggers	"Stress" triggers
	Usually no pain syndrome	Chronic pain
	Later refractory	Unresponsive to multiple drugs
Ictus	Eyes open	Eyes closed
	Short duration	Long duration
	Typical tonic or tonic–clonic	Asynchronous (stop–start–stop)
	Nonpurposeful	May be purposeful
	No response to voice	Turns head when called
	Oxygen desaturation	No oxygen desaturation
	Dysautonomia	No dysautonomia
Postictus	Breathing heavily	Normal breathing
	Lactic acidosis	Normal ABG
	CPK elevated	Normal CPK
	Prolactin elevated	Normal prolactin
	Tongue bite (lateral)	Tongue bite (tip)

ABG = arterial blood gas; CPK = creatine phosphokinase.

usefulness. In a recent study, only 3% of patients in the ED with suspected seizures had EEG confirmation after extended EEG monitoring, but also included patients with prior epilepsy.[12]

In Practice

For any emergency room physician, it is important to recognize that ictal symptoms can cause falls and injury, that the attacks are associated with complete loss of consciousness, and that this may last for over several minutes. Most of the time, the clonic phase is 2–3 minutes and wanes gradually. Some of these attacks may include chewing, smacking, licking, or any other automatisms. Some patients only have picking at sheets or fumbling movements of the arms. Again, the eyes are mostly open during a generalized tonic–clonic seizure, and the head turns to one side, also with eye deviation. The mouth is tightly shut. The patient is flushed in his face and should not show a bluish skin or lip unless there is evidence of aspiration and desaturation. Emergency physicians are guided by recent recommendations of the American College of Emergency Physicians. Many emergency physicians would define the type of seizure first, followed by dividing it into provoked versus unprovoked seizure. An acute symptomatic seizure has been arbitrarily defined as occurring within 7 days from a systemic, toxic, or metabolic derangement or occurring in an evolving CNS lesion. Unprovoked seizures are those without a cause. Epilepsy may result from recurrent unprovoked seizures, but could be a result of a static neurologic lesion (arteriovenous malformation, mesial temporal lobe epilepsy, hamartoma). Current guidelines call for no antiepileptic drugs for first provoked seizure or first unprovoked seizure without a brain lesion. Antiepileptic drugs should be strongly considered in patients with a first unprovoked seizure and remote history of brain lesion (e.g., prior stroke, prior trauma, or brain surgery).[10] Recurrence after first unprovoked seizure is 20%–45% in first 2 years. Risk is highest in patients with prior brain lesions, abnormal EEG, and nocturnal seizures.[15] More than 90% of these patients stay seizure-free on low to moderate doses of a variety of antiepileptic drugs.[13] Side effects can remain very low with these low doses.[20] Patients who have fully recovered from a first unprovoked seizure do not necessarily need to be admitted if neurologic examination is not concerning and CT is unremarkable.[10] However, the threshold for admission should be low. It allows observation of the patient follow-up CPK levels, which can more or less unexpectedly rise to the 10,000s. An prolonged EEG can be obtained. In one study, epileptiform activity was found in 20% of admitted patients.[8]

Treatment of seizures is indicated in Table 6.4. The question is how much clinical management is allowed or permitted in the ED. A single seizure can be treated with

Table 6.4 **Initial Treatment Options of Seizures**

Drug	*Dose*	*Adverse Effects*
Phenytoin	18–20 mg/kg administered no faster than 50 mg/kg; increase to total 30 mg/kg if seizures continue	Soft-tissue injury with extravasation, hypotension, cardiac dysrhythmias, purple glove syndrome
Fosphenytoin	18–20 PE/kg administered no faster than 150 PE/min	Hypotension, cardiac dysrhythmias
Valproate	20–30 mg/kg at rate of 40 mg/min	Dizziness, thrombocytopenia, liver toxicity, hyperammonemia
Levetiracetam	30–50 mg/kg IV load at 100 mg/min	Nausea, rash
Propofol	2 mg/kg; may repeat in 3–5 min; maintenance infusion of 25–100 mcg/kg/min	Injection site pain, heart failure, respiratory support required
Midazolam	0.2 mg/kg load and maintenance infusion 0.75 mcg/kg/min	Hypotension
Pentobarbital	10–20 mg/kg; maintenance infusion of 1 mg/kg/h	Respiratory depression, hypotension

PE = phenytoin equivalent; IV = intravenous.

4–8 mg of lorazepam, followed by 20 mg/kg of (fos)phenytoin infusion. Any patient who has a secondary seizure should be admitted emergently to an ICU, preferably an NICU for EEG monitoring and further treatment that often will include an anesthetic drug. Not every patient with a single seizure will have to be admitted to an ICU; however, two seizures—even of short duration—would likely require a brief observation in a monitored setting because the chance of a third seizure is high. A CT scan is indicated in every patient. A lumbar puncture is indicated if the patient is febrile or if there is a high suspicion of a CNS infection. It is important to recognize that herpes simplex encephalitis can present with a single generalized tonic–clonic seizure before confusion or any other focal findings. Seizures in bacterial meningitis are uncommon as a first presentation; other clinical symptoms are far more apparent, such as decreased level of consciousness, neck stiffness, and evidence of a febrile response.

Psychogenic nonepileptic seizures are common, and the cost per patient in the United States is approximately $100,000 per patient per year.[16] Psychogenic nonepileptic seizure is possibly the preferred term, but it has also been known as conversion response, pseudoseizure, or psychogenic seizure. There are many unusual descriptions that can be helpful in determining these nonepileptic seizures. Often, the motor activity is bizarre and includes pelvic thrusting, hyperextension, flailing, or thrashing. Most noticeable is that patients may have a purposeful movement such as grasping the bedrail or the examiner. Most importantly, after this event, the patient has a good recollection of what happened. For the emergency physician, there are several pitfalls. Failure to recognize a nonepileptic seizure may lead to aggressive management that is unnecessary, potentially causing iatrogenic complications. Conversely, inaccurate diagnosis of nonepileptic seizures while the patient does have frontal lobe epilepsy or myoclonic or temporal lobe epilepsy is equally important, although many of those seizures can be recognized after further workup following admission. No patient should be dismissed from the ED until seen by a neurologist or admitted briefly for further evaluation. This may be direct admission to an epilepsy monitoring unit that would require a video EEG.[24]

It is highly uncertain whether induction protocols are useful in the ED, although simple treatments might be useful. Compression of the temple region, massaging it with a finger after explaining that it could induce the event, appears to have a high sensitivity (65%) and a high specificity (100%). Torchlight stimulation, moist swab application, tuning fork application, or—even worse—saline injection have much less possibility of inducing a seizure. A suggestion to the patient to prepare the "especially large needle that may induce a seizure" is inappropriate and deceitful.[3] Induction protocols are usually preferred in a more monitored setting.[9] Justification for these induction tests is that they could avoid inappropriate treatment exposing the patient to unnecessary drug toxicity. However, one could argue that these provocative tests are better performed during a video EEG monitoring, documenting an unchanged EEG. (Detection of motion artifact during video monitoring can be difficult to detect in some patients, although the absence of postictal slowing may help distinguish artifact from clinically significant EEG changes.) Psychogenic nonepileptic status epilepticus has been reported in several instances and the movements are very different. The most useful clinical test, apart from finding that eyes are closed, is to find inability to perform an oculocephalic reflex. Patients with nonepileptic seizures cannot voluntarily generate roving eye movement, and the oculocephalic reflex is an uninhibited reflex that should be absent. Using cold water flushing in the ear to obtain an ocular vestibular response is inappropriate, definitively unprofessional, and perhaps also unethical due to the high incidence of vomiting and possible aspiration. Psychogenic status epilepticus is recognized by several clinical signs.[4] Flailing arms, shaking in two extremities alone (often alternating), hip thrusts, and rolling movement are common features. Up to 60% of the patients with pseudoseizures meet *Diagnostic and Statistical Manual of Mental Disorders* criteria for a personality disorder.

Patients should be offered comprehensive treatment with a neuropsychologist or a psychiatrist and a social work or a rehabilitation consultant.[14] The best strategy is to explain to the patient that antiepileptic drugs are not effective and that it is not epilepsy and to explain that precipitating factors are related to stress or emotions. It is important to avoid the terms "hysterical seizures". Some have argued that even the word "seizure" should be avoided.

EEG is helpful if done immediately in the ED. Serum prolactin has been used in the past and could differentiate between true seizure and pseudoseizure, because the level is elevated in a true seizure when measured 10–20 minutes after the event. The test—serum value peaks briefly—is rarely used in clinical practice and is often not elevated in status epilepticus.

What about management of the other spells? The ED is not the proper place to further differentiate the type of the spell; patients need to be temporarily admitted to a monitored bed. This will allow recognition and better description of the spell assuming it repeats itself. Documentation that it is a true syncope or documentation of a cardiac arrhythmia may be possible (Chapter 3). Further testing for unusual causes may be rewarding. Any patient with a spell and a fall needs admission after an orienting trauma evaluation for fractures.

TRIAGE

In many situations, a brief observation in the ED is sufficient to provide guidance for further evaluation in the clinic. If there is more than one spell, the patient should be admitted to a monitored bed. If there is one single seizure and no evidence (CT scan, laboratory tests, or possibly CSF) of a new neurologic problem, the patient can be dismissed. Seizure recurrence is substantial in a patient with a new-onset seizure and demonstrable brain lesion and thus requires antiepileptic therapy and admission.

Putting It All Together

- Seizures occur in patients prone to get seizures.
- The decision to treat a seizure with medication depends on the presence of a brain lesion.

- Seizures do not necessarily require intubation and "bagging" will suffice.
- Seizures may cause very significant laboratory abnormalities.
- Spells and pseudoseizures are common in the ED.
- Pseudoseizures are unfortunately often treated with antiepileptic drugs.

By the Way

- A third of patients on antiepileptics have breakthrough seizures.
- Most people who have a seizure do not end up with epilepsy.
- Early outcome is determined by the presence of acute brain lesion.
- Labored breathing is what bystanders remember after a seizure.
- Aspiration is common, but chest X-ray often clears rapidly.

Seizures and Nonepileptic Seizures by the Numbers

- ~25% of patients with pseudoseizures become seizure free.
- ~25% of patients with a seizure in the ED will receive neuroimaging.
- ~25% of patients with pseudoseizures have prior diagnosis of epilepsy.
- ~20% of patients with a seizure seen in the ED are admitted.
- ~10% of pseudoseizures have a precipitating life event.
- ~1% of all ED visits are for seizures.

References

1. Abdel Baki SG, Omurtag A, Fenton AA, Zehtabchi S. The new wave: time to bring EEG to the emergency department. *Int J Emerg Med* 2011;4:36.
2. Angus-Leppan H. First seizures in adults. *BMJ* 2014;348:g2470.
3. Burton JL. "Pseudo" status epilepticus. *Lancet* 1989;2:632.
4. Cervenka MC, Lesser R, Tran TT, et al. Does the teddy bear sign predict psychogenic non-epileptic seizures? *Epilepsy Behav* 2013;28:217–220.
5. Engel J, Jr. *Seizures and Epilepsy*. Vol 83. New York: Oxford University Press; 2012.
6. Fernandez IS, Loddenkemper T, Datta A, et al. Electroencephalography in the pediatric emergency department: when is it most useful? *J Child Neurol* 2014;29:475–482.
7. Firosh Khan S, Ashalatha R, Thomas SV, Sarma PS. Emergent EEG is helpful in neurology critical care practice. *Clin Neurophysiol* 2005;116:2454–2459.
8. Goldberg I, Neufeld MY, Auriel E, Gandelman-Marton R. Utility of hospitalization following a first unprovoked seizure. *Acta Neurol Scand* 2013;128:61–64.
9. Goyal G, Kalita J, Misra UK. Utility of different seizure induction protocols in psychogenic nonepileptic seizures. *Epilepsy Res* 2014;108:1120–1127.
10. Huff JS, Melnick ER, Tomaszewski CA, et al. Clinical policy: critical issues in the evaluation and management of adult patients presenting to the emergency department with seizures. *Ann Emerg Med* 2014;63:437–447 e415.
11. Jordan KG. Continuous EEG monitoring in the neuroscience intensive care unit and emergency department. *J Clin Neurophysiol* 1999;16:14–39.
12. Kadambi P. Hart K, Adeoye OM, et al. Electroencephalopgraphic findings in patients presenting to the ED for the evaluation of seizures. *Am J Emerg Med* 2015;33:100–113.
13. Kwan P, Brodie MJ. Effectiveness of first antiepileptic drug. *Epilepsia* 2001;42:1255–1260.

14. LaFrance WC, Jr., Reuber M, Goldstein LH. Management of psychogenic nonepileptic seizures. *Epilepsia* 2013;54 Suppl 1:53–67.
15. Krumholz A, Wiebe S, Gronseth GS, et al. Evidence-based guideline: management of an unprovoked first seizure in adults. *Neurology* 2015;84:1705–1713.
16. Martin R, Bell B, Hermann B. Nonepileptic seizures and their costs: the role of neuropsychology. In: Prigatano GP, Pliskin NH, eds. *Clinical Neuropsychology and Cost Outcome Research: A Beginning*. New York: Psychology Press; 2003:235–258.
17. McKenzie P, Oto M, Russell A, Pelosi A, Duncan R. Early outcomes and predictors in 260 patients with psychogenic nonepileptic attacks. *Neurology* 2010;74:64–69.
18. Noble AJ, Goldstein LH, Seed P, Glucksman E, Ridsdale L. Characteristics of people with epilepsy who attend emergency departments: prospective study of metropolitan hospital attendees. *Epilepsia* 2012;53:1820–1828.
19. Pallin DJ, Goldstein JN, Moussally JS, et al. Seizure visits in US emergency departments: epidemiology and potential disparities in care. *Int J Emerg Med* 2008;1:97–105.
20. Perucca P, Jacoby A, Marson AG, et al. Adverse antiepileptic drug effects in new-onset seizures: a case-control study. *Neurology* 2011;76:273–279.
21. Praline J, Grujic J, Corcia P, et al. Emergent EEG in clinical practice. *Clin Neurophysiol* 2007;118:2149–2155.
22. Privitera MD, Strawsburg RH. Electroencephalographic monitoring in the emergency department. *Emerg Med Clin North Am* 1994;12:1089–1100.
23. Schmidt D, Schachter SC. Drug treatment of epilepsy in adults. *BMJ* 2014;348:g254.
24. Siket MS, Merchant RC. Psychogenic seizures: a review and description of pitfalls in their acute diagnosis and management in the emergency department. *Emerg Med Clin North Am* 2011;29:73–81.
25. Young WF, Jr., Maddox DE. Spells: in search of a cause. *Mayo Clin Proc* 1995;70:757–765.
26. Zaidi A, Clough P, Cooper P, Scheepers B, Fitzpatrick AP. Misdiagnosis of epilepsy: many seizure-like attacks have a cardiovascular cause. *J Am Coll Cardiol* 2000;36:181–184.

7

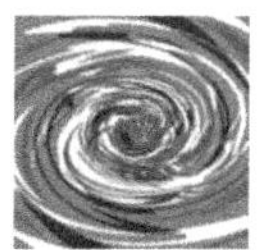

Triaging Traumatic Brain and Spine Injury

Traumatic brain and spine injury mostly involves patients who have had motor vehicle accidents, have been assaulted, or have fallen, some from significant heights. Depending on the impact, polytrauma may occur and much of it is clearly visible. Arrival at the ED triggers a Level I trauma alert that focuses all attention toward the patient rescue. Initially, the medical complexities of these highly unstable patients are largely in the hands of the emergency room physician and trauma surgeon. The priority is to manage chest and abdominal trauma in multitraumatized patients, taking precedence over the management of TBI. Acute chest or abdominal exploration for injury has priority often due to its immediate life-threatening condition. In addition, there may be complicated decisions pertaining to timing of fixation or instrumentation of long-bone fractures.

A pertinent issue for many emergency healthcare workers is to know what to expect from the neurologist and for the neurologist to know how to contribute. Because traumatic brain and spine injury is so common and so complex, this series of six books on core principles in acute neurology has four chapters on the topic of TBI. Each chapter provides a situational approach. This chapter focuses on immediate triage and stabilization of the most severely affected patient and what role a consulting neurologist could and must play. It also concentrates on which elements of assessment are prone to be missed or underrecognized. Judging the severity of any type of TBI and initial care is discussed in the volume *Handling Difficult Situations*. Several other major neurologic complications with polytrauma besides TBI are discussed in the volume *Solving Critical Consults*. Prognosis of TBI is found in the volume *Communicating Prognosis* and discusses the major CRASH and IMPACT outcome calculators.

New information has shown that, according to the US CDC, TBI has increased by 20%.[7] It remains a major neurologic and neurosurgical problem.[16,23,29] Most of what is seen arriving in the ED are motor vehicle accidents. In addition, there might be an additional effect of intoxication with alcohol or IV drug use. This means that these patients—mostly young men—will have more severe injuries. Some drugged patients are found on the street or in the recesses of buildings, often in a deplorable clinical condition.

No question the problem of care of TBI starts way outside the hospital and whether direct access to a trauma center can be achieved. Transfer to a trauma center in a patient with an acute epidural or acute subdural hematoma is mandatory. Access to a trauma center with a step in between may harm the patient. However, whether outcomes in TBI can be improved with quick transfer to a trauma center is unclear.[10,18] Several studies have found that increased lactate level (or slow clearance on repeat studies), need for transfusion (several units of blood), emergency chest tubes, and laparotomy predict early demise.[22] In contrast, the ability to successfully intubate a patient before hospital transfer improves outcome.[28] Moreover, treatment of coagulopathy in the CRASH-2 study markedly improved outcome.[25]

When the neurologist becomes involved with acute traumatic brain and spine injury—directly or as intermediary or facilitator—the questions that will likely be asked the following: Is the clinical presentation fitting with the neuroimaging study? Are the CT scans appropriately read? What findings on CT scan are particularly worrisome? Are the spine X-rays ordered and appropriately read? Is there possibly increased ICP that needs treatment? Is there sufficient attention to avoidance of secondary injury due to systemic factors? Do we immediately need a neurosurgeon?[2–4] These important issues should come up early in triage of these severely injured patients.

Principles

There are specific areas of interest to the neurologist. First, of course, evaluation starts with a neurologic examination, but it is more specialized and specific.

One of the first core principles is to document the essential findings on examination. It is often embarrassing for neurologists to note that neurologic examination is either not done or consists of a GCS (the omnipresent 3T, see Chapter 2). As expected, the most important neurologic finding in any comatose patient with a TBI is dilated pupils fixed to light. The presence of one or two unreactive dilated pupils and extensor posturing is significantly associated with unfavorable outcome and these have been robust indicators in many large databases.[14,15] In fact, of all factors used in prognostication, these two simple findings are the most important to record. As alluded to in Chapter 2, a detailed examination of other key brainstem reflexes is crucial in further determining severity of TBI. Examination should include further characterization of the pupil size (oval, midposition, small), presence of anisocoria, corneal reflexes, oculovestibular reflexes (not oculocephalic reflexes that require neck movements), facial mimicry to pain, cough response to suctioning, and breathing type or triggering of the ventilator. It is almost inexcusable that several of these findings are not recorded in TBI studies, usually as a result of overreliance of the GCS. Some combinations of absent brainstem reflexes are very worrisome, and this assessment may be helpful to triage and determines action.

Neurologists and neurosurgeons immediately recognize that in a patient with an acute hemorrhagic contusion or a large epidural or subdural hematoma, a unilateral fixed dilated pupil is a neurosurgical indication because it will be followed by bilateral fixed pupils, and that changes the equation quickly. Neurologists and neurosurgeons also recognize that bilateral fixed pupils with absence of some other brainstem reflexes and evidence of axonal brain injury with early brain swelling bode poorly for a satisfactory outcome. Neurologists and neurosurgeons also recognize that prognostication in young individuals with TBI is fraught with errors because many can bounce back over a year.

The second core principle is to look for other warning signs in TBI. There are some immediate potential issues to attend to. In the midst of multiple trauma to limbs, abdomen, or chest, the presence of facial trauma may receive less attention. Paradoxically, neurologists may be the first to point out scalp and facial injuries. Scalp avulsions may cause significant blood loss and should be repaired immediately. In a few instances, hypotension may result from major external scalp bleeding. Most likely hypotension in TBI has been caused by hypovolemia due to inadequate fluid resuscitation, use of osmotic agents, hyperglycemia-induced osmotic diuresis, cold diuresis, or diuresis as a result of sudden rewarming. If no cause for hypotension is obvious, the neurologist is often asked for a possible neurologic explanation. Definitively uncommon but a known fact is that hypotension in young children may occur with a large, epidural hematoma. In adults, the answer to this question is simple: Hypotension in adults is rarely a direct result of TBI unless the patient has progressed and has become brain dead. Loss of the sympathoexcitatory neurons in the rostroventrolateral medulla cause loss of vascular tone. Hypotension may occur with severe spinal cord injury. In patients with a marked spinal cord injury or a severed spinal cord, the circulation becomes fragile also due to loss of sympathetic tone. Hypotension may become profound from vasodilatation. The typical finding in these spinal cord injuries is warm extremities but marked hypotension from redistribution to the peripheral circulation.

Most important are abrasions of the chin and they may be tell tale signs of a retroflexion movement causing trauma to the cervical spine and a cervical collar should be placed without delay, until a cervical spine imaging has excluded a fracture or dislocation and the neck has been "cleared". A recent review found that CT of cervical spine is an appropriate and sufficient test.[1] Orbital swelling can be profound and may prevent full examination of fundi and eye movements. If the swelling is associated with ecchymosis of the eyelids (the so-called raccoon or panda bear eyes), it may indicate a fracture of the orbital roof or, more commonly, a Le Fort III (nasal-orbital-ethmoid midface) or zygomatic fracture. The orbital roof fracture may extend through the ethmoid or cribriform–ethmoid junction and result in a CSF fistula. Petrous bone fractures may result in facial paralysis from direct injury to the facial nerve, ecchymosis over the mastoid (Battle's sign), and a CSF leak. (The Battle and raccoon eye signs, however, take hours to develop, and specificity for basal skull fracture is low.)

The third core principle is to expect seizures—overt or subtle—in patients with TBI. Clinical seizures are seen in only up to 10% of patients with TBI and are more common in patients with a traumatic intracerebral hematoma, depressed skull fracture, and a dural tear. There is some evidence that alcohol-related TBI (mostly patients with prior alcohol abuse) could increase the chance for seizures. Continuous EEG monitoring has been able to point to many more subtle seizures and may be needed particularly after an emergent evacuation of a subdural hematoma compressing the cortex. In transferred patients, it is helpful to instruct the nursing staff in the ED to look for subtle signs of seizures (staring, eye deviation, facial and eyelid twitching), which if present should lead to EEG recording and treatment. Early focal (or generalized) seizures can be very persistent, and aggressive control even with double coverage of 2 g IV levetiracetam and fosphenytoin 20 mg/kg IV infusion may be needed for the first few days, followed by a change to monotherapy and preferably levetiracetam for at least 1 month—a period when seizures are most common. Levetiracetam has the best safety profile of all antiepileptic drugs and levetiracetam may have additional neuroprotective properties in acute brain injury.[12,31] Treatment of EEG abnormalities alone has not resulted in improving the outcome, so these abnormalities may be nothing more than markers of cortical injury (contusion) or irritation (traumatic SAH). Seizures should be differentiated from early vigorous shivering and posturing as a result of paroxysmal sympathetic hyperactivity syndrome ("autonomic storming"). Dysautonomia may appear quite early after TBI and on the same day, but if so, it indicates a severe diffuse axonal brain injury. Patients clench both fists, bury the thumbs into the palms; grind teeth; lock the jaw; and bite the endotracheal tube—all with profuse sweating and tachycardia.

Once the patient is neurologically and medically stable, a decision will have to be made based on the type and urgency of the TBI. There are several important severity indicators of TBI, and they are shown in Table 7.1. Many of them involve the type of injury, age, and whether there are systemic factors such as tachypnea or hypotension.

Several classifications have been developed that help in focusing care.[19,21] One simply classifies the severity of TBI on the basis of the type of injury—closed, penetrating—and whether there is a parenchymal or extraparenchymal hematoma. (There is a larger definitional problem with mild brain injury.[19]) Subsequently, an effort is made to identify skull fractures, particularly those that might be depressed and require immediate assessment by neurosurgery for the exploration of an associated dural tear. Basilar skull fractures may be associated with vascular lacerations, particularly carotid artery trauma. (For a detailed discussion on traumatic vascular injury see the volume *Solving Critical Consults.*)

Table 7.1 **Severity Indicators of Traumatic Brain Injury**

Inability to remember trauma
Fall, fist fight, car collision
Age >60 years
Tachypnea
Hypotension
Scalp or face injury
Penetrating injury
Pupils fixed to light
Abnormal findings on computed tomographic scan

Another way to assess the severity is to categorize patients according to the severity of injury including confounding factors such as intoxication or presence of anticoagulation. This so-called BIG (brain injury guidelines) classification is helpful in focusing attention and triage and is shown in Table 7.2. It has been used to define the management of TBI by acute care surgeons, who often are present in large trauma centers. It also arguably defines the need for repeat CT and neurosurgical consultation. Interestingly, one study with more than 1,000 patients with TBI and abnormal CT scan findings found that these patients' categories related to clinical or radiological worsening. Neurosurgical intervention was most often seen in BIG 3 but not in BIG 1 or BIG 2.[12]

Medical management and observation in extracerebral hematomas are considered only for alert patients with no worsening and generally mild motor deficit. Epidural or subdural hematomas with a diameter less than 4 mm, no midline shift, and no lucent area inside the hematoma suggesting recent bleeding could be managed with observation (Figure 7.1). For subdural hematomas, medical management is considered if the thickness of the hematoma is similar to the thickness of the skull. Subdural hematomas without any shift (caused by atrophy of the brain in elderly patients or chronic alcoholics) can be surgically managed in a delayed fashion when the clinical signs are

Table 7.2 **Brain Injury Guidelines (BIG)**

Variables	*BIG 1*	*BIG 2*	*BIG 3*
LOC	Yes/No	Yes/No	Yes/No
Neurologic examination	Normal	Normal	Abnormal
Intoxication	No	No/Yes	No/Yes
CAMP	No	No	Yes
Skull Fracture	No	Nondisplaced	Displaced
SDH	≤4 mm	5–7 mm	≥8 mm
EDH	≤4 mm	5–7 mm	≥8 mm
IPH	≤4 mm, 1 location	3–7 mm, 2 locations	≥8 mm, multiple locations
SAH	Trace	Localized	Scattered
IVH	No	No	Yes
Therapeutic Plan			
Hospitalization	No observation (6 h)	Yes	Yes
RHCT	No	No	Yes
NSC	No	No	Yes

CAMP = coumadin, aspirin, plavix; EDH = epidural hemorrhage; IVH = intraventricular hemorrhage; IPH = intraparenchymal hemorrhage; LOC = loss of consciousness; NSC = neurosurgical consultation; RHCT = repeat head computed tomography; SAH = subarachnoid hemorrhage; SDH = subdural hemorrhage.

Source: From Joseph et al.[12]

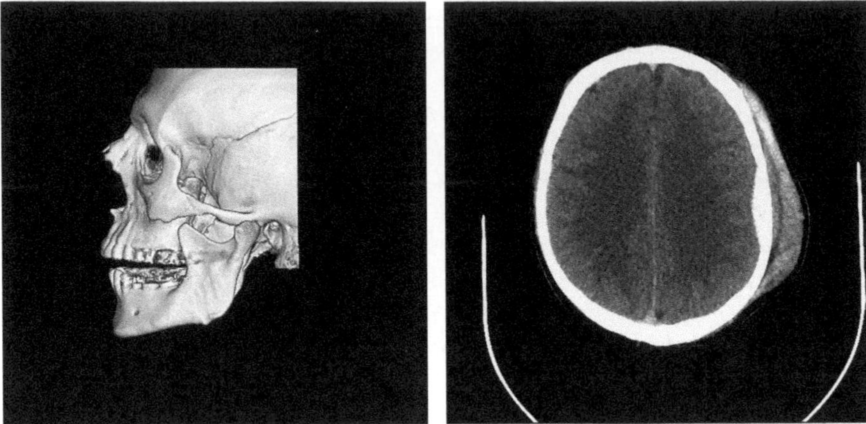

Figure 7.1 Parietal Bone Fracture with Epidural Hematoma.

minimal. Surgical management of extracerebral hematomas may be urgently indicated, but there has been a significant downward trend in surgical procedures without negatively affecting outcome.[9]

In Practice

Physicians in the ED will identify the immediate priorities in TBI (Table 7.3). Without sounding too intuitive, this includes securing the airway, removing a foreign body, intubating endotracheal with fiberoptic gliding device to avoid any neck movement, and inserting venous catheters. It is important to provide fluids with

Table 7.3 **Immediate Priorities in Severe Traumatic Head Injury**

Secure airway
Remove foreign body
Endotracheal intubation
Immobilize spine
Secure venous access with two catheters
Inspect for scalp laceration and depressed fracture
Stat CT chest, abdomen, pelvis with hypotension
Obtain cervical spine X-ray or CT cervical spine
Chest radiography (or repeat)
CT scan of brain (or repeat)

CT=computed tomography.

two large-bore catheters. A trauma patient who fails to respond to fluid therapy, with no obvious bleeding source in the chest, and no fractures should be presumed to have bleeding in the abdomen until proved otherwise. Abdominal ultrasound sonography may find fluid in the peritoneal cavity and is highly sensitive, but many patient will undergo an urgent CT of chest, abdomen, and pelvis.

There is a reasonable consensus about the standards of fluid management in TBI and what the targets are. Some experts argue for a flat body position to maximize cerebral perfusion pressure (CPP), and that should be considered if the blood pressures are soft. Early fluid resuscitation in an attempt to improve organ and brain perfusion is beneficial. Others have argued that fluid administration may reduce blood viscosity and dilute clotting factors. Administration of poorly warmed fluids may also contribute to a coagulopathy. A consensus approach consists of guarded fluid resuscitation, correction of any hypothermia, and use of vasopressors if needed. In any patient, transfusion of red blood cells (1 unit for each 1 g decline) is needed if hemoglobin is less than 8 g/dL.

Hypoxemia should be aggressively managed, and after intubation, increasing positive end-expiratory pressure (PEEP) may be needed to improve gas exchange. PEEP may increase intrapleural pressure and superior vena cava pressure and reduce cerebral venous outflow. ICP may become seriously elevated if PEEP values higher than 10 cm H_2O are needed, but its increase can be countered with mannitol and head elevation. Also, PEEP may increase SAH $PaCO_2$ because of increased physiologic dead space; this effect should be anticipated and managed by increasing the minute volume of the ventilator. The correctable causes of increased ICP are shown in Table 7.4.

Rapid triage to CT is essential, because it determines the cause of impaired consciousness in most instances.

The next priority is to evaluate neuroimaging. Unfortunately, there is a need for better recognition and quantification of injuries to the brain after TBI. A recent study found a poor inter-rater reliability between emergency room physicians when asked to classify the type of injury. When CT scans are shown with subdural hematomas, epidural hematomas, SAH, contusion, or diffuse axonal injury, the agreement between emergency physicians leaves much to be desired, indicating a need to have CT scans evaluated by a neuroradiologist, a neurologist, a neurointensivist, or a neurosurgeon.[13] It should be pointed out that MRI is underutilized and may show additional

Table 7.4 **Correctable Causes of Increased Intracranial Pressure**

- Surgical evacuation of cerebral or extracerebral hematoma
- Drainage of trapped ventricles with ventriculostomy
- Aggressive control of seizures with IV antiepileptics
- Improve oxygenation with PEEP or change in oxygen flow
- Reduce coughing, straining, and pain with IV fentanyl
- Treat abdominal distension (surgery or nasogastric tube on suction)
- Treat fever aggressively with cooling device

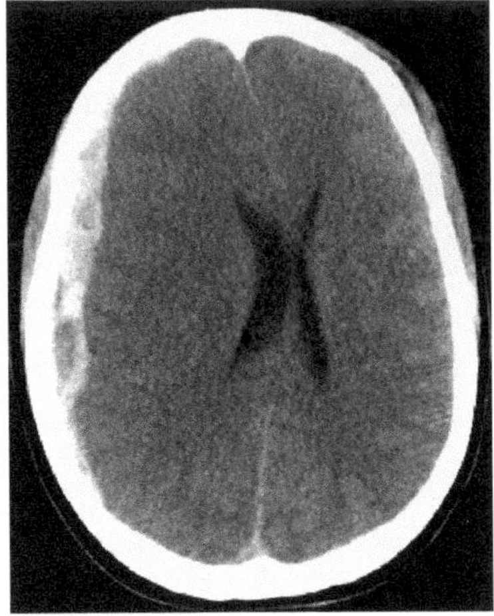
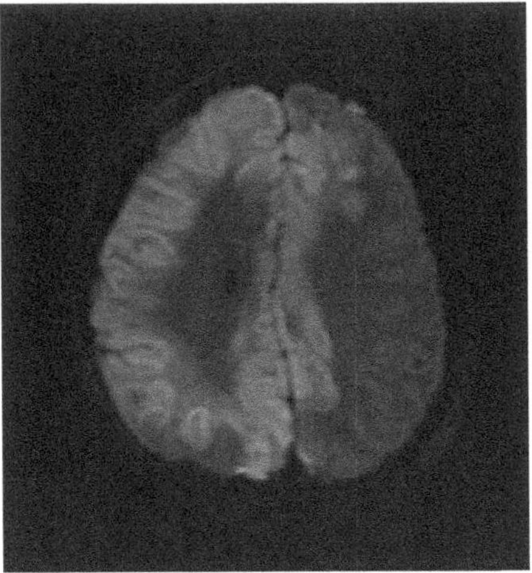

Figure 7.2 Evacuation of acute subdural hematoma and no clinical improvement explained by severe anoxic-ischemic injury on MRI.

anoxic-ischemic brain injury in patients with TBI who do not recover after a craniotomy (Figure 7.2).

Again, the main principle of management of traumatic head injury is immediate treatment of a presumed ICP, which may involve removal of an extracranial hematoma or contusion with mass effect. ICP monitoring has traditionally been considered in many comatose patients after TBI; but a recent trial—comparing clinical judgment and CT interpretation with decisions based on ICP values—found no difference in outcome. In other words, aggressive management of patients with "presumed increased ICP" is not better than management based on ICP values from ICP monitors.[5] Furthermore, a recent study found that ICP monitoring occurred in less than half of the patients who were eligible (14 trauma centers during a 2-year study period).[6] In this important study, the patients who underwent ICP monitor placement were younger and lower-risk surgical candidates with more significant intracranial injuries. ICP monitoring resulted in reduced mortality. Older patients and patients with coagulopathy received less often ICP monitors. Thus, decisions on who received ICP monitors is somewhat arbitrary and often based on ad-hoc risk assessment by the neurosurgeon.

The focus of management involves not only reduction of ICP but also maintenance of an interrelated cerebral perfusion pressure (CPP) and mean arterial pressure (MAP). The abbreviated formula defining the relationship is CPP=MAP-ICP. In addition, it is important to recognize that vasodilatation and vasoconstriction cascades may exist (Figure 7.3). These cascades are important in identifying the role of CPP. Cerebral blood flow is held constant within the range of mean arterial pressure from 80 to 160 mm Hg. Outside this range, cerebral blood flow is linearly coupled with pressure. Below the lower threshold, a decrease in CPP results in a decrease in blood flow and ischemia. Theoretically, above the upper threshold, an increase in CPP results in breakdown of the blood–brain barrier and edema, but studies suggest that high perfusion pressures are tolerated for brief periods. Management of CPP has been advocated, but it

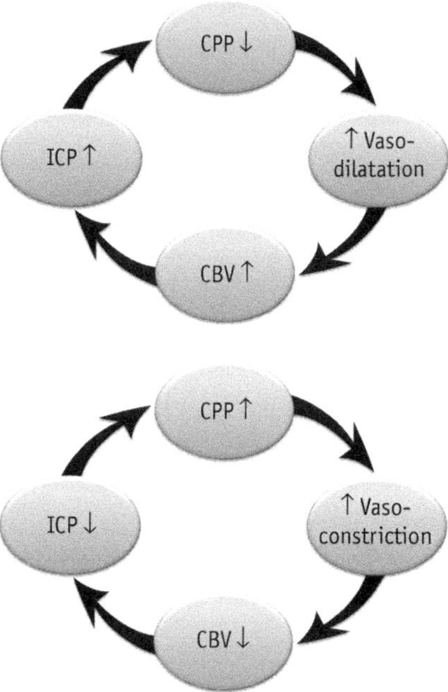

Figure 7.3 Relationships between intracranial pressure (ICP),cerebral perfusion pressure (CPP) and cerebral blood volume (CBV).

assumes intact autoregulation, which may not be present in up to 50% of patients with severe TBI. Cerebral perfusion is usually aimed at 70–80 mm Hg and can be increased by increasing systolic arterial blood pressure, draining CSF pressure, and using mannitol. These vasodilatory and vasoconstriction cascades have led to the management of CPP irrespective of ICP. Blood pressure can be increased with vasopressors and normovolemia is maintained with albumin. However, adequate preservation of CCP is only useful if there is coexisting treatment of ICP. Cerebral perfusion can be increased by increasing systolic arterial blood pressure, draining CSF pressure, or using osmotic agents.

If there is a suspicion of increased ICP on CT (basal cisterns compressed, midline shift, several hemorrhagic contusions, and a potential surgical lesion, it is prudent to hyperventilate the patient (frequency of more than 20 breaths/minute or squeezing the anesthesia [Ambu] bag every 3 seconds) and to give a single loading dose of mannitol (20%), 1 g/kg over 10 minutes, but only if blood pressure has remained stable throughout. A restless intubated patient may require sedation with propofol (infusion of 0.5 mg/kg/h) or dexmedetomidine (0.4–1.5 mcg/kg/h). When there is significant dysautonomic storming, meperidine (0.4 mg/kg IV every 4 hours) can be administered. These paroxysms are also best aggressively treated with a cooling blanket.

Several simple measures also reduce ICP, such as preventing head rotation to one side (jugular vein compression); suctioning without stimulation of the soft palate or posterior pharyngeal wall, which elicits a gag and cough reflex; and suctioning through an endotracheal tube limiting to one passage only. IV administration of lidocaine or lidocaine spray or increasing the dose of propofol may blunt these ICP responses. Several drugs may potentially increase ICP through an increase in cerebral blood flow by vasodilation and should be avoided (e.g., hydralazine, sodium nitroprusside, ketamine, and nicardipine).

In many patients, one of the priorities is to provide immediate hyperosmolar therapy. Care in the ED is variable when surveyed.[26] In a recent study with emergency physicians in Level II trauma centers, half of emergency room physicians used hypertonic saline, and most used hypertonic saline in the presence of severe TBI with unilateral unreactive pupils, midline shift, or cistern compression. Most neurologists will first administer 20% mannitol 1 g/kg infusion. In patients with hypotension, hypertonic saline (3% or 10%) can be used, but a rapid bolus of 30 cc (23% hypertonic saline) may cause hypotension due to sudden peripheral vasodilation.

Over the years, a stepwise model has emerged to treat ICP. The steps are likely as follows: increased sedation, ventricular drainage, hyperosmolar therapy, induced hypocapnia, hypothermia, barbiturates, and as a last resort decompressive craniectomy. Many experts argue against a protocol-driven approach. Some have argued for better understanding of the pathophysiology and to achieve that through multimodal brain monitoring.

Admission to a Level I trauma center improves mortality rates.[17] Mortality is four times higher with no transfer to a Level I trauma center, also known as "undertriage."[20] Several clinical signs and CT scan findings are important, and outcome triangles are shown in Figure 7.4. These findings are not absolutes, but they may drive management (they certainly are used to exclude patients from clinical trials). In TBI, outcome is determined mostly at onset, but major management issues remain that include management of dysautonomia; bladder, skin, and bowel care; and planning for stabilization.

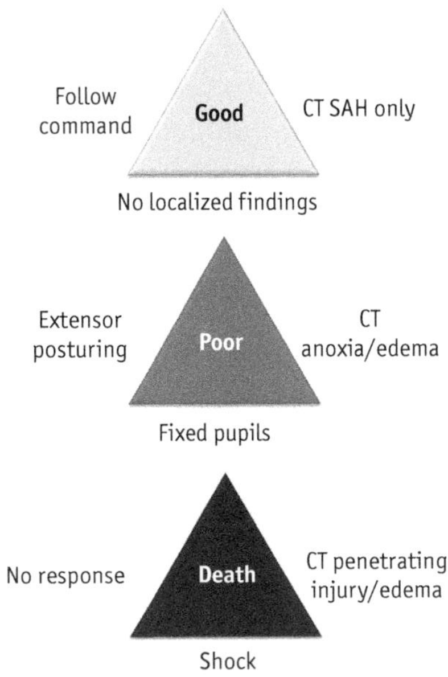

Figure 7.4 Outcome triads for traumatic brain injury.

Table 7.5 **Emergency Room Management of Traumatic Spine Injury**

Intubation and mechanical ventilation with lesion at C3 or higher
Intubate if aspiration
Volume loading with albumin or Ringer's lactated solution
Epinephrine drip
Body warming with blanket, warming intravenous fluids
Subcutaneous heparin, or early consideration of IVC filter.
Codeine for pain
Proton pump inhibitor to prevent gastrointestinal bleeding
Interval 0–3 h methylprednisolone 30 mg/kg
Infusion of methylprednisolone 5.4 mg/kg/h for 24 h
Interval 3–8 h methylprednisolone 30 mg/kg
Infusion of methylprednisolone 5.4 mg/kg/h for 48 h

An equally complicated situation is to recognize and stabilize spinal injury. Stabilizing spinal surgery is often needed.[8,30] MRI scans would indicate further injury to the spine, but in most situations, the clinical examination determines management. A patient with a complete cervical transection and apnea unavoidably need to be intubated, and most of these patients are tetraplegic. Patients with a transection above C3 cannot be weaned.[27]

The initial emergency room management of traumatic spine injury is shown in Table 7.5.

The use of methylprednisolone has been questioned, but most patients will receive methylprednisolone infusion if seen within a certain time limit. Most of the injury is determined by using the American Spinal Injury Association Impairment Scale. Surgical decompression for acute spinal cord injury is highly debated, and whether early decompression may benefit outcome is completely unclear. The early versus delayed decompression for traumatic cervical spine injury study (Surgical Timing in Acute Spinal Cord Injury Study: STASCIS) has found some benefit in neurologic outcome and intensive care complications. However, this clinical trial has not led to a consensus to what might be the best approach.[8,30]

TRIAGE

The triage of a TBI should be toward the operating room in patients who have an epidural or subdural hematoma or hemorrhagic contusional mass, particularly if there is a progressive decrease in consciousness, hemiparesis, or a speech deficit.[18,24] Placement of ICP monitor and monitoring in NICU is mandatory in many ICU centers. All patients with traumatic spine injury need first medical stabilization before spine surgery. Spine trauma requires evaluation of specialized orthopedic surgeons and neurosurgeons.

Putting It All Together

- Triage and admission to a Level I trauma center should provide best options for survival.
- Secondary transfer to Level I trauma is associated with fourfold increase in mortality.
- Early attempts at ICP management are warranted and ICP does not have to be known.
- Not all contusions need ICP management.

- Certain CT categories predict severity of injury and risk of deterioration.
- Not all subdural hematomas need immediate neurosurgical intervention.
- Spinal cord injury requires multidisciplinary evaluation and early intervention.

By the Way

- Bias against salvageability of patients determines transfer to trauma center.
- Availability of neurosurgeon determines outcome of extracerebral hematoma.
- Control of coagulopathy determines outcome of TBI.
- Concurrent lesions of brain and spine injuries affect mostly C1-C4 injury.

Triaging Traumatic Head and Spine Injury by the Numbers

- ~75% of patients reach Level I trauma center for definitive care.
- ~50% of patients with TBI receive an ICP monitor.
- ~25% of patients with severe trauma have dual spine and brain injuries.
- ~25% of patients with unilateral fixed pupil have a good outcome.
- ~20% of patients with TBI have continuously normal ICP readings.

References

1. Badhiwala JH, Lai CK, Alhazzani W, et al. Cervical spine clearance in obtunded patients after blunt traumatic injury: a systematic review. *Ann Intern Med* 2015;162:429–37.
2. Bratton SL, Chestnut RM, Ghajar J, et al. Guidelines for the management of severe traumatic brain injury. XI. Anesthetics, analgesics, and sedatives. *J Neurotrauma* 2007;24 Suppl 1:S71–76.
3. Bratton SL, Chestnut RM, Ghajar J, et al. Guidelines for the management of severe traumatic brain injury. XIV. Hyperventilation. *J Neurotrauma* 2007;24 Suppl 1:S87–90.
4. Carney NA. Guidelines for the management of severe traumatic brain injury: methods. *J Neurotrauma* 2007;24 Suppl 1:S3–6.
5. Chesnut RM, Petroni G, Rondina C. Intracranial-pressure monitoring in traumatic brain injury. *N Engl J Med* 2013;368:1751–1752.
6. Dawes AJ1, Sacks GD, Cryer HG, et al. Intracranial pressure monitoring and inpatient mortality in severe traumatic brain injury: A propensity score-matched analysis. *J Trauma Acute Care Surg* 2015;783:492–502.
7. Faul M, Xu L, Wald MM, Coronado VG. *Traumatic Brain Injury in the United States: Emergency Department Visits, Hospitalizations and Deaths 2002–2006*. Atlanta, GA: Centers for Disease Control and Prevention, National Center for Injury Prevention and Control; 2010.
8. Fehlings MG, Vaccaro A, Wilson JR, et al. Early versus delayed decompression for traumatic cervical spinal cord injury: results of the Surgical Timing in Acute Spinal Cord Injury Study (STASCIS). *PLoS One* 2012;7:e32037.
9. Flynn-O'Brien KT, Fawcett VJ, Nixon ZA, et al. Temporal trends in surgical intervention for severe traumatic brain injury caused by extra-axial hemorrhage, 1995–2102. *Neurosurgery* 2015;76:451–460.

10. Fuller G, Lawrence T, Woodford M, Coats T, Lecky F. Emergency medical services interval and mortality in significant head injury: a retrospective cohort study. *Eur J Emerg Med* 2015;22:42–48.
11. Joseph B, Friese RS, Sadoun M, et al. The BIG (brain injury guidelines) project: defining the management of traumatic brain injury by acute care surgeons. *J Trauma Acute Care Surg* 2014;76:965–969.
12. Kirmani BF, Mungall D, Ling G. Role of intravenous levetiracetam in seizure prophylaxis of severe traumatic brain injury patients. *Front Neurol* 2013;4:170.
13. Laalo JP, Kurki TJ, Sonninen PH, Tenovuo OS. Reliability of diagnosis of traumatic brain injury by computed tomography in the acute phase. *J Neurotrauma* 2009;26:2169–2178.
14. Maas AI, Murray GD, Roozenbeek B, et al. Advancing care for traumatic brain injury: findings from the IMPACT studies and perspectives on future research. *Lancet Neurol* 2013;12:1200–1210.
15. Maas AI, Steyerberg EW, Marmarou A, et al. IMPACT recommendations for improving the design and analysis of clinical trials in moderate to severe traumatic brain injury. *Neurotherapeutics* 2010;7:127–134.
16. Maas AI, Stocchetti N, Bullock R. Moderate and severe traumatic brain injury in adults. *Lancet Neurol* 2008;7:728–741.
17. MacKenzie EJ, Rivara FP, Jurkovich GJ, et al. A national evaluation of the effect of trauma-center care on mortality. *N Engl J Med* 2006;354:366–378.
18. Mejaddam AY, Elmer J, Sideris AC, et al. Prolonged emergency department length of stay is not associated with worse outcomes in traumatic brain injury. *J Emerg Med* 2013;45:384–391.
19. Menon DK, Schwab K, Wright DW, Maas AI. Position statement: definition of traumatic brain injury. *Arch Phys Med Rehabil* 2010;91:1637–1640.
20. Nirula R, Maier R, Moore E, Sperry J, Gentilello L. Scoop and run to the trauma center or stay and play at the local hospital: hospital transfer's effect on mortality. *J Trauma* 2010;69:595–599.
21. Okie S. Traumatic brain injury in the war zone. *N Engl J Med* 2005;352:2043–2047.
22. Regnier MA, Raux M, Le Manach Y, et al. Prognostic significance of blood lactate and lactate clearance in trauma patients. *Anesthesiology* 2012;117:1276–1288.
23. Roozenbeek B, Maas AI, Menon DK. Changing patterns in the epidemiology of traumatic brain injury. *Nat Rev Neurol* 2013;9:231–236.
24. Rosenfeld JV, Maas AI, Bragge P, et al. Early management of severe traumatic brain injury. *Lancet* 2012;380:1088–1098.
25. Shakur H, Roberts I, Bautista R, et al. Effects of tranexamic acid on death, vascular occlusive events, and blood transfusion in trauma patients with significant haemorrhage (CRASH-2): a randomised, placebo-controlled trial. *Lancet* 2010;376:23–32.
26. Sharma S, Gomez D, de Mestral C, et al. Emergency access to neurosurgical care for patients with traumatic brain injury. *J Am Coll Surg* 2014;218:51–57.
27. Stein DM, Roddy V, Marx J, Smith WS, Weingart SD. Emergency neurological life support: traumatic spine injury. *Neurocrit Care* 2012;17 Suppl 1:S102–111.
28. Stiell IG, Spaite DW, Field B, et al. Advanced life support for out-of-hospital respiratory distress. *N Engl J Med* 2007;356:2156–2164.
29. Thompson HJ, McCormick WC, Kagan SH. Traumatic brain injury in older adults: epidemiology, outcomes, and future implications. *J Am Geriatr Soc* 2006;54:1590–1595.
30. van Middendorp JJ, Hosman AJ, Doi SA. The effects of the timing of spinal surgery after traumatic spinal cord injury: a systematic review and meta-analysis. *J Neurotrauma* 2013;30:1781–1794.
31. Zafar SN, Khan AA, Ghauri AA, Shamim MS. Phenytoin versus Leviteracetam for seizure prophylaxis after brain injury—a meta analysis. *BMC Neurol* 2012;12:30.

8

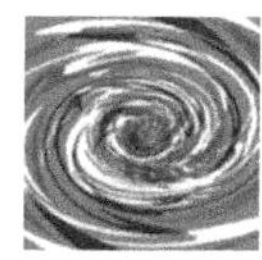

Triaging Acute Ischemic and Hemorrhagic Stroke

It is remarkable that a considerable number of patients with an acute stroke do not seek urgent medical help.[12] Given the acute changing nature of stroke, it may be surprising that delay is so common. But if patients with an acute stroke do get where they belong, EDs have treatments and protocols in place to respond quickly. Most of the time any new acute hemiparesis, a language or speech problem prompts a "stroke call," which involves a blast text page, alerting emergency room physicians, designated stroke neurologists, hospitalists or neurointensivists, stroke or neurointensive care fellows, the pharmacist, and most importantly radiologists and technicians operating machinery that can provide a miscellany of neuroimaging. Acute stroke calls cast a wide net, but even then only a fraction of all patients with suspicious signs will jump through the necessary hoops to get acute intervention. Such calls can be effective if it can be demonstrated that as a result very few patients with acute stroke slip through. Acute stroke call usually involves ischemic and hemorrhagic strokes, but does not necessarily exclude SAH or traumatic cerebral hemorrhage. The emergence of Teleneurology is changing the landscape rapidly. Telestroke improves diagnostic accuracy and improves decision making.

To break it down to the most essential tasks, the major involvement for neurologists in the ED is to decide when to proceed with IV tPA in ischemic stroke and then to find specific entry criteria for endovascular intervention to retrieve a clot in a proximal cerebral artery occlusion. In patients with intracranial hemorrhage (ICH), there are multiple initial considerations, but in the first hours, it is all about securing airway, correction of a coagulopathy, and management of a concerning hypertensive surge. There is no question that deteriorating patients with superficially located lobar hematoma may need to be acutely sent to the operating room.

What goes on in the ED is the main focus of this chapter. There is a golden hour in the management of acute stroke when decisions must be made quickly. The following questions can be asked: Who is eligible for IV tPA and what are the current contraindications? When can we assume the patient does not respond to IV tPA? At what point do we alert the neurointervention team? Which cerebral hemorrhages are the most unstable? Can we reliably predict expansion of cerebral hemorrhage? How can we best neurologically stabilize an intracranial hemorrhage? These pieces of information are needed to adequately triage patients with an acute ischemic or hemorrhagic stroke.

Principles

In stroke, certain patterns and syndromes have become recognized, and thus part of the principles of management in acute stroke is also recogniting these acute stroke syndromes. Each of them has specific concerns and urgent decisions, with the ultimate goal being to minimize the damaged territory, because reducing the infarct size or stabilizing the clot size increases the chance of a favorable clinical outcome.

STROKE AND THE EMERGENCY DEPARTMENT

The improved technology, particularly 4G technology, results in stable cellular networks and stable Internet connection and allows robots and cameras in both distant EDs and ambulances. There is now good information not only about the feasibility and logistics of telemedicine but also on the possible impact on outcome. A handful of studies have been performed, of which two were in the United States, that showed variable results but also technical failure and more concerning the inability to perform not more than a third of the Telestroke consultations but this will improve significantly if it has not already.[4,20–23,32,33] A well-run Telestroke program will increase the use of tPA, simply because many emergency physicians feel uncomfortable giving IV tPA without a neurologic consultation.[29] Telestroke visits may evaluate not only ischemic stroke but also when a CT scan is much different, and thus may change management of SAH and evaluation of lobar of ganglionic cerebral hematomas. Of course, seeing these patients with Telestroke programs creates not-to-be-missed opportunities, and there is a good chance care will be more thought through. Neurologists can provide help with decisions on use of osmotic agents in shifted intracranial hematomas, when to seek emergency neurosurgical evaluation in the same hospital for early placement of a ventriculostomy, or evacuation of an hematoma or when to transport to a closer hospital rather than undertaking a long trip. Most of the time, however, Telestroke referral networks connect with communities with no stroke management capabilities. Increased use of thrombolysis should theoretically improve functional outcome, because thrombolysis is effective, but only 5% of patients with ischemic stroke receive this intervention. Moreover, it appears that thrombolysis is not used in incapacitated patients who cannot make decisions and who have no surrogate decision-makers available. (When asked, a recent study found, in elderly patients—here defined as more than 50 years old—a large proportion is interested in thrombolysis if they were to be in that situation.[8])

Another novel strategy is the involvement of a mobile stroke unit and installation of a CT scanner in the ambulance.[10] Initial trial runs have shown that it is feasible with stable technology signals and that only 10 minutes of consultation are needed to make the decision to use tPA. If this can be established worldwide, the impact on stroke care can be revolutionary, assuming the patient gets in the ambulance in time.

ASSESSMENT OF ISCHEMIC STROKE

The first core principle is that one should recognize an ischemic stroke quickly. That may seem trite to say, yet some studies have found that of patients who were initially diagnosed with an ischemic stroke, 60% had other conditions.[27] After the diagnosis is made and consent for IV tPa is obtained, the time-to-needle interval is important. This time interval may improve in an environment that allows Telestroke, but a real paradigm shift will be when stroke neurologists are easily available. To reach these critical benchmarks requires a multiplicity of protocols and pathways that lead to adequate disposition and transfer. Several studies have found that there are strategies to reduce the stroke onset-to-treatment time through not only targeted education campaigns but also transfer to a stroke center by EMS and prenotification of hospitals by EMS, rapid triage protocol, the so-called all-points-alarm activation system, rapid laboratory testing, and rapid access to IV-administered tPA, which includes the availability of tPA in an ED. More recently, strategies have included the patient bypassing the ED and transporting the patient directly to the CT suite, where IV tPA is administered to eligible patients after performance and interpretation of a noncontrast CT scan. There is sufficient evidence that prehospital triage to primary stroke centers improves the use of tPA, in fact doubles IV tPA use at primary stroke centers.[26] Most studies have found that directly going to the CT scanner is the step where most gains are made if these protocols are used.[24] Data from the United States has shown that before aggressive prenotification protocols, only 30% of door-to-needle time was less than 1 hour.[26] In general, the average door-to-needle time in the United States is approximately 72 minutes and over the recommended treatment within 60 minutes on arrival.

There are several time points and several opportunities for improvement (Figure 8.1). It is a major logistical problem to improve the door-to-needle time. Some countries are exemplary (Finland), when logistics are in place and the result is a door-to-needle time within 20 minutes. There is some hyperbole. Some have cleverly argued that for every minute of treatment delay, there is a loss of nearly 2 million neurons.[28] But to say, "it is simply unacceptable not to achieve very fast treatment" ignores the common failure of any physician to recognize stroke, failure to act on a stroke, and failure to change a basic human behavior to be slow to act in a crisis.[17]

The second core principle is to recognize atypical presentations of acute cerebrovascular syndromes. These include an acute confusional state or altered level of consciousness in a thalamic stroke, an acute movement disorder associated with a stroke in the basal ganglia, and seizures, although they are more likely to occur in patients with a stroke associated with cerebral sinus thrombosis.[11] The National Institutes of Health Stroke Scale (NIHSS) is not able to recognize strokes in the posterior circulation that present with vertigo or marked gait difficulties, and it does not specifically recognize most of the cognitive abnormalities that may include anosognosia or

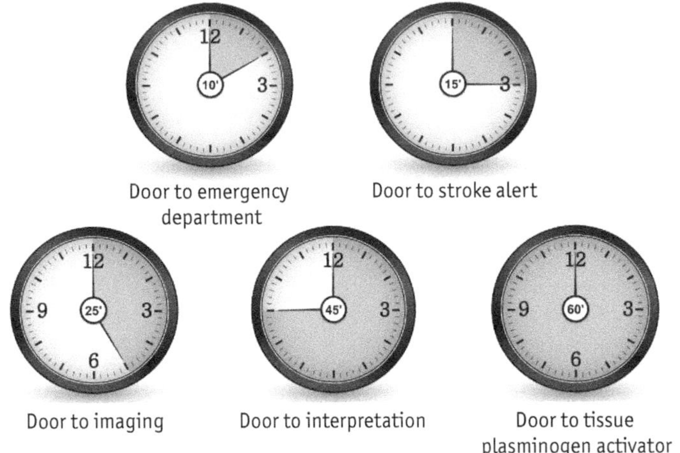

Figure 8.1 Time to thrombolysis.

aprosodia. Several types of ischemic strokes, particularly if they involve the caudate nucleus or frontal lobe, can present with neurobehavioral problems rather than focal findings.

tPA catalyzes plasmin formation from plasminogen, and plasmin degrades circulatory fibrinogen and the fibrin lattice of the thrombin into soluble end products. Tissue plasminogen activator decreases or depletes measurable circulating plasminogen and fibrinogen and results in a prolongation of the partial thromboplastin time. Alteplase is the currently used IV thrombolytic, but tenecteplase is more potent and has advantages of a rapid single bolus, but there is insufficient evidence of superiority or noninferiority as compared with alteplase. A recent comparative study showed no difference in effect, but tenecteplase was administered on average 20 minutes faster than alteplase.[18]

tPA is often inappropriately deferred in patients with mild but disabling deficits. Prior use of aspirin, prior strokes, and old age have been considered risks for hemorrhage complications. A recent task force reevaluated the eligibility of thrombolysis. Their consensus regarding eligibility based on disabling neurologic deficits is shown in Table 8.1.

The third core principle is therefore to rapidly find reasons to give IV thrombolytics and not to hesitate but also not to err too much toward the side of caution. If there is one opportunity to improve disability in ischemic stroke early and hours after onset, it is IV thrombolysis.[18] IV thrombolysis can be started if there are no clinical contraindications, no radiographic contraindications—usually with evidence of an ICH or a large territorial stroke—or a laboratory contraindication with a prothrombin time of more than 15 seconds, INR more than 1.7, platelet count of less than 100.000/L, and a blood glucose level of less than 50 mg/dL. Moderate hyperglycemia is not a

Table 8.1 **Disabling Neurologic Deficits**

Complete hemianopsia (≥2 on the NIHSS question 3)
Severe aphasia (≥2 on NIHSS question 9)
Visual or sensory extinction (≥1 on NIHSS question 11)
Any weakness limiting sustained effort against gravity (≥2 on NIHSS question 5 or 6)
Any deficits that lead to a total NIHSS > 5
Any remaining deficit considered potentially disabling in the view of the patient and the treating practitioner (Clinical judgment required)

contraindication, but when there is extreme hyperglycemia and metabolic acidosis (i.e., 600–800 mg/dL), signs such as severe dysarthria or aphasia may appear, mimicking acute stroke. Recent surgery is an exclusion criterion but when surgery involves body areas that can be easily amenable to hemostasis, thrombolysis should not be deferred. This remains a gray area; these types of surgeries may involve recent thoracentesis or other biopsy procedures.

In general, IV thrombolysis tPA can be started within 3–4.5 hours of onset unless there is major resolution of symptoms. Usually, IV tPA is administered using 0.9 mg/kg but with a 90 mg maximum. Administration is with a 10% bolus in 1-minute injection and 90% of the total drug in 1-hour infusion. When patients are seen beyond the 4.5–6-hour window with a stroke in the anterior cerebral circulation and NIHSS >8, endovascular treatment should be considered. There is a longer time of treatment opportunity in the posterior cerebral circulation (Figure 8.2).

CTA and perfusion (or MRA and perfusion MRI) can be performed if there are profound motor, language, and sensory deficits with eye deviation, all pointing to a major intracranial vessel occlusion. This pertains to a clot location in the MCA M1 or proximal M2 (sylvian fissure) branch. In the posterior circulation, many patients have developed new eye findings (anisoria, skew deviation), motor deficits (quadriparesis), or acute coma with extensor motor responses. Endovascular treatment involves removal of the embolus in the basilar artery or proximal branching with the posterior cerebral artery. Endovascular retrieval of clot has been shown to improve outcome in five recent clinical trials. Stent retrieval has been used predominantly, but the ultimate goal is rapid recanalization and the method is secondary. The clinical trials have been able to achieve a perfusion close to 4 hours after onset at best.[14] (More details on how these decisions are made are discussed in, *Handling Difficult Situations*).

Major logistical problems remain and rapid access to centers with immediate endovascular availability remains limited. It is only for a few patients because the number of patients with proximal artery occlusion and still preserved brain tissue who will be eligible for clot retrieval may be as low as 1% of all ischemic strokes.[5,7] But if there is a small infarct core and moderate-to-good collateral circulation, outcome definitively improves in these patients. Referrals to endovascular centers will increase over the years.

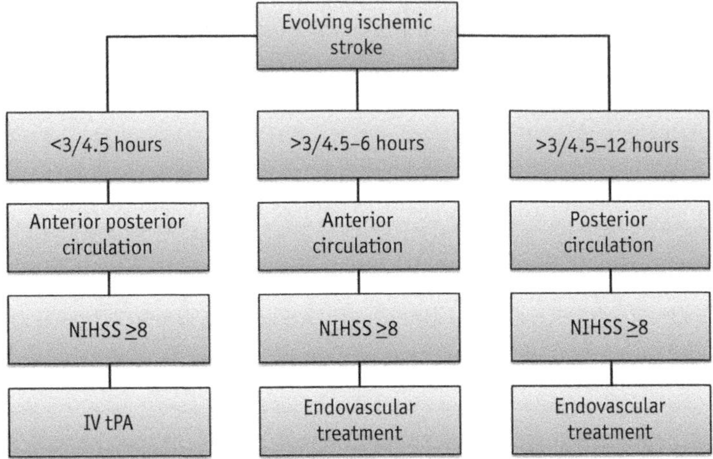

Figure 8.2 Treatment in acute ischemic stroke.

The third core principle is to carefully manage blood pressure in patients eligible for IV thrombolysis. There remains uncertainty about the goals of care and which blood pressure–lowering medication to use. The AHA/ASA guideline suggests a target of blood pressure of less than 180/110 mm Hg at start of tPA administration and less than 180/105 mm Hg in the first 24 hours after tPA administration. Without use of tPA, antihypertensives should be held to allow for "permissive hypertension." Such "permissiveness" may include systolic blood pressures up to 220 mm Hg or a mean blood pressure of up to 120 mm Hg. Neither of these recommendations is supported by strong evidence and the correlation between hypertension and post IV thrombolysis or post clot retrieval hemorrhage is not firmly established.

INTRACRANIAL HEMORRHAGE

Several guidelines have been published, but again, many are based on expert opinion and low quality of evidence.[1,30,31] The major priorities in ICH are the prediction of hematoma growth, management of blood pressure, and correction of coagulopathy, mostly warfarin-associated ICH.

The fourth core principle involves the determination of intracranial volume that involves the use of the ABC-2 method. This calculates the volume on a CT image. This ellipsoid volume method measures the largest hemorrhage on a slice, maximal length (A) and the diameter perpendicular to this line (B), and the number of slices multiplied by the slice thickness (C). This allows estimation of ICH volume in cubic centimeters.

The ICH score is currently used in many accredited comprehensive stroke centers and is shown in Table 8.2. This score forces the physician to obtain a level of consciousness, measure a volume, note the presence of intraventricular hemorrhage—whether it is infratentorial or supratentorial—and obtain an age that combine to indicate the initial prognosis assessment. The score is simple and does not identify many other important clinical features such as new brainstem findings, neither does it identify CT scan features such as shift nor the development of acute hydrocephalus from ventricular trapping that may require ventriculostomy. It has nothing to say about risk factors for extension of volume.

Cerebral hematomas are usually a consequence of long-standing hypertension, but one study of over 600 patients with ICH found detectable vascular lesions in 17% (9% arteriovenous malformation, 3% aneurysm, 2% cerebral venous thrombosis, 1% Moya Moya, and 2% arterial or venous malformation). Thus, there may be a reason to proceed with a CTA in the ED.[19] These are typically patients with temporal lobe and sylvian fissure clots suggesting a ruptured aneurysm. Any young patient with no known risk factors for cerebral hemorrhage may harbor an aneurysm, an arteriovenous malformation, or a dural arteriovenous fistula. CTA and may also detect contrast extravasation within the clot (spot sign)—roughly in a third of the patients seen within 10 hours of presentation and is highly (80%) predictive of subsequent hematoma expansion

Table 8.2 **Determining the ICH Score**

Component	*ICH Score points*
Glasgow Coma Scale (GCS)	
3–4	2
5–12	1
13–15	0
ICH volume (mL)	
≥30	1
<30	0
Intraventricular hemorrhage	
Yes	1
No	0
Infratentorial origin of ICH	
Yes	1
No	0
Age (years)	
≥80	1
<80	0
Total ICH score	0–6

Notes: ICH volume on initial CT calculated using ABC/2 method. GCS score is on initial presentation (or after resuscitation). ICH = intracerebral hemorrhage.

Source: From Clarke et al.[9] and Hemphill et al.[15]

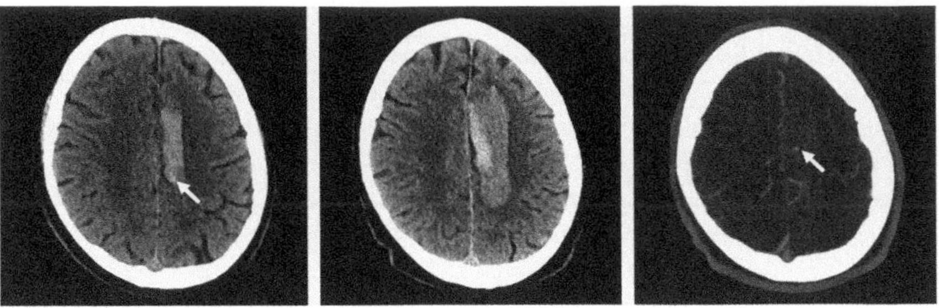

Figure 8.3 The spot sign in cerebral hemorrhage.

(Figure 8.3). However, several other pieces of information may predict expansion. This includes the time to initial CT scan and the size of the hemorrhage.[6] Hematoma growth is expected when

$$\frac{\text{Baseline ICH volume}}{\text{Time onset to CT}} > 10 \text{ mL/h}$$

Studies may investigate the clinical effect of rapid INR correction in the presence of such a sign. CTA in the ED however is rarely used and hard to defend outside a clinical trial.[19]

A fifth core principle is to act immediately in reversing anticoagulation, whatever its cause (Table 8.3). Warfarin-related ICHs enlarge quickly (Figure 8.4) and are best treated with PCC. Fresh frozen plasma contains 1–2 units of each clotting factor and fibrinogen per milliliter. The INR of fresh frozen plasma is about 1.3. Fresh frozen plasma rarely rapidly corrects INR. Prothrombin complex is a collection of factor concentrates that is separated from large plasma pools and then reconstituted. These products contain vitamin K–dependent factors; factors II, VII, IX, and X; and proteins C and S. (The 3 factor PCC contains little factor VII, the 4 factor PCC contains normal amounts of factor VII. It is unknown if there are significant differences, but 4 factor PCC is more often used with extreme high INR's). The major benefit of prothrombin complex is that it is 25% less

Table 8.3 **Options in Anticoagulation Reversal**

Warfarin	Vitamin K: 10 mg IV Prothrombin complex concentrate: 20–50 IU/kg Factor VIIa: 10–20 mcg/kg Fresh frozen plasma: 15 mL/kg
Heparin	Protamine: 1 mg/100 units of heparin (maximal dose of 50 mg)
LMWH	Protamine and prothrombin complex concentrate
tPA	Tranexamic acid: 1 g and 1 hour infusing 10 mg/kg IV Cryoprecipitate: 0.15 IU/kg (repeat if fibrinogen <100 mg/dL)
Thrombin and factor Xa inhibitors	Prothrombin complex concentrate: 20 IU/kg Hemodialysis

LMWH = low-molecular-weight heparin; tPA = tissue plasminogen activator; IV = intravenous.

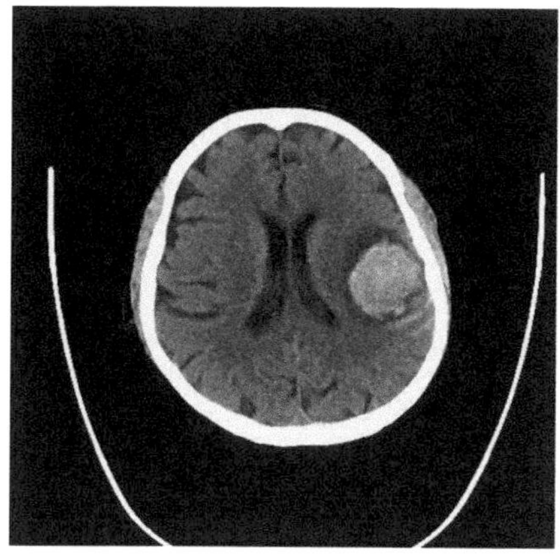
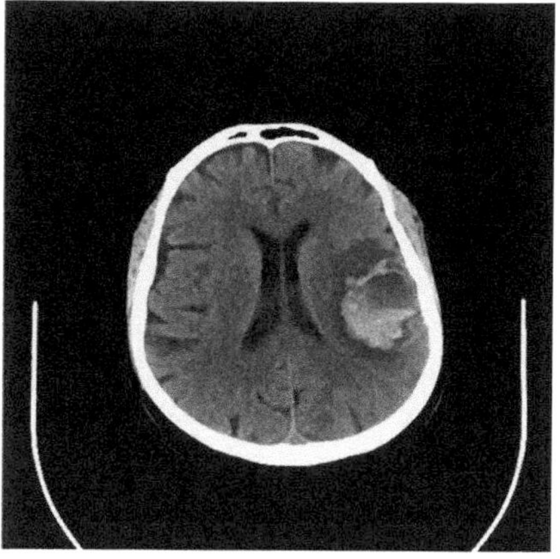

Figure 8.4 Warfarin associated lobar hematoma (note fluid level).

volume than fresh frozen plasma and thus decreases the likelihood of fluid overload. Often PCC is a slow IV infusion with a rate not exceeding 2 mL/min. The INR is repeated after infusion and then every 6 hours over the first 24 hours, with new PCC infusions if the INR rebounds. Target INR is ≤ 1.3 and this value would allow any neurosurgical intervention if necessary. An example of dose adjustment dependent on starting INR is shown in Table 8.4. Several large studies have found that PCC not only faster corrects INR than fresh frozen plasma but also has fewer adverse effects and therefore should be the first line of treatment.[16]

If the hemorrhage occurs while the patient is on IV heparin, one should immediately administer 1 mg of protamine sulfate for every 100 IU of active heparin. In low-molecular-weight heparin, protamine is administered, along with a factor VIa or PCC. There is, unfortunately, no antidote for fondaparinux. There are similar problems with direct thrombin inhibitors and direct factor Xa inhibitors. Fortunately, the half-life of these drugs is short, but there is no specific reversal agent. There is little that can be done with the thrombin inhibitors, and hemodialysis has been proposed next to PCC.[2,13]

A crucial decision is whether to use platelet transfusion in patients with an ICH. Platelet transfusion with one pack (6 units of platelets) results in improved platelet

Table 8.4 **Example of Calculation of Dose of Factor IX Complex**

INR	*Dose*
>5	55 IU/kg
>4	50 IU/kg
>3	45 IU/kg
>2	40 IU/kg
>1.5	20 IU/kg

activity.[25] Inhibition is reversed in approximately 65% of patients with platelet transfusion, but two-thirds of initial nonresponders were corrected after a second transfusion.[3] Clinically it remains unclear whether the best approach is to give two transfusions but we do when there has been prior use of dual antiplatelet agents. However, no study has shown that there is any mortality benefit or improved functional outcome with platelet transfusion in patients with ICH who were on antiplatelet medication. In patients with thrombocytopenia, platelet transfusions are very necessary and one transfusion often brings platelet counts up to the 70,000 level. This may apply to patients with liver cirrhosis, acute leukemias, or other major hematologic malignancies, but despite improvement in platelet counts hemorrhage may still progress.

The sixth core principle is to control hypertension. Current guidelines do not establish a target, although the American Heart Association suggests reducing blood pressure to less than 160–190 mm Hg or mean arterial blood pressure to less than 110 mm Hg. If ICP is also monitored, a CPP of more than 60 mm Hg should be maintained. This is only in patients in which a ventriculostomy has been placed due to acute obstructive hydrocephalus and a small proportion of patients with ICH.

The seventh core principle is to consider early evacuation of the hematoma. Triaging to surgery is generally advised if the patient is deteriorating and if tissue shift is seen on CT scan. Worsening and enlargement of the hematoma must prompt surgical management, even if major clinical trials in stable patients have not found a difference in outcome. Trials in deteriorating patients have not been performed and surgery in these patients may be most beneficial. (A detailed discussion is found in the *Handling Difficult Situations.*)

In Practice

Initial management of an acute ischemic stroke in the ED is to protect the airway with endotracheal intubation if desaturation has occurred. Some patients with a large territorial stroke may have aspirated and may desaturate. In general, it is important to avoid any antihypertensive medication and to accept a mean arterial blood pressure of less than 130 mm Hg and to allow "permissive hypertension". Many patients will need to be immediately rehydrated with 0.9% saline using 2 L at least in the first 24 hours, and hyperglycemia should be corrected, maintaining a glucose between 140 and 180 mg/dL. Temperature control is important, although most of the patients will develop fever after the first 24 hours and it does not appear to be an issue in the ED.

Massive acute hemispheric infarction—particularly in patients with acute carotid artery occlusion—is often fatal once cerebral edema develops. In large cerebellar infarctions, neuroimaging and serial neurologic assessments can be used to distinguish between altered level of consciousness from hydrocephalus or direct brainstem compression. Such a distinction can help with selection of the most appropriate therapy (ventricular drainage versus surgical decompression) targeted to the underlying mechanism.

Early decompressive craniectomy can be considered in large ischemic strokes with brain tissue shift. The procedure is commonly refused by family members and mostly performed in younger individuals. Concerns about major morbidity in survivors have been voiced, and the functional outcome in elderly patients is marginal. On the other hand, with a cerebellar infarct and swelling, many patients eventually become independent after decompressive surgery.[34]

The decision to proceed with surgical evacuation in a large cerebral hematoma remains difficult. Any comatose patient with a large-volume ganglionic hematoma or lobar hematoma will likely deteriorate within hours after admission and show a fixed and dilated pupil despite measures to reduce mass effect, such as osmotic agents. We have seen patients with lobar hematoma and early signs of clinical and radiological brainstem compression who recovered well after emergency evacuation of the hematoma. Timing of surgery in most patients is unknown, but most neurosurgeons proceed with the first signs of deterioration. Ganglionic hematomas do not benefit from evacuation via a traditional open craniotomy that requires dissecting through healthy brain tissue. Expectedly, surgery in comatose patients with a cerebral hematoma was ineffective in large clinical trials.

Patients who are in need of urgent surgery are those with a vascular anomaly (such as an arteriovenous malformation, a large cavernous hemangioma, or an aneurysm). Because of the risk of recurrent hemorrhage soon after initial presentation. Surgery also performed in patients in whom there is suspicion of an underlying tumor.

Another neurosurgical issue is the placement of a ventriculostomy in a patient with cerebral hematoma and obstructive hydrocephalus. This intervention may result in clinical improvement.

TRIAGE

The most important decision is to get a patient with an ischemic or an hemorrhagic stroke out of the ED. This can be best accomplished with well-run policies: whom to call and page, how to get a neurosurgeon quickly, and how to get the patient to the necessary neuroimaging that determines the practical next step. Triage to an ICU (or NICU) is needed, but some patients need to go to interventional radiology suite (large vessel occlusion and major hemispheric syndrome) or operating room (lobar hematoma with shift).

Putting It All Together

- Too many patients with a stroke do not seek help, or get help too late.
- Quick access to IV thrombolytics remains a phenomenal challenge.
- Major benefit of telestroke programs is that it increases the frequency of thrombolytic administration.
- Blood pressure control and anticoagulation reversal before hospital arrival is the best option for successful outcome in cerebral hematoma.

- Immediate reversal of anticoagulation is needed and before any transport.
- Expansion of the cerebral hematoma may increase mortality.

By the Way

- Stroke alerts have put neurologists on alert and with success.
- Transport should be with fastest means.
- Heads-up on arriving patients will reduce time to needle.
- Heads-up on possible endovascular treatment may reduce time to recanalization.

Triaging Ischemic and Hemorrhagic Stroke by the Numbers

- ~80% recanalization can be achieved with endovascular therapy.
- ~40% of patients with demonstrable recanalization have good outcome.
- ~30% of patients with acute stroke do not call for help within 1 hour.
- ~15% of patients with a cerebral hemorrhage may have a vascular lesion.
- ~5% of patients with a cerebral hemorrhage need reversal of anticoagulation.

References

1. Aguilar MI, Hart RG, Kase CS, et al. Treatment of warfarin-associated intracerebral hemorrhage: literature review and expert opinion. *Mayo Clin Proc* 2007;82:82–92.
2. Awad AJ, Walcott BP, Stapleton CJ, et al. Dabigatran, intracranial hemorrhage, and the neurosurgeon. *Neurosurg Focus* 2013;34:E7.
3. Bachelani AM, Bautz JT, Sperry JL, et al. Assessment of platelet transfusion for reversal of aspirin after traumatic brain injury. *Surgery* 2011;150:836–843.
4. Bergrath S, Reich A, Rossaint R, et al. Feasibility of prehospital teleconsultation in acute stroke—a pilot study in clinical routine. *PLoS One* 2012;7:e36796.
5. Berkhemer OA, Fransen PS, Beumer D, et al. A randomized trial of intraarterial treatment for acute ischemic stroke. *New Engl J Med* 2015;372: 11–20.
6. Brouwers HB, Chang Y, Falcone GJ, et al. Predicting hematoma expansion after primary intracerebral hemorrhage. *JAMA Neurol* 2014;71:158–164.
7. Campbell BC, Mitchell PJ, Kleinig TJ, et al. Endovascular therapy for ischemic stroke with perfusion-imaging selection *New Engl J Med* 2015;372:1009–1018.
8. Chiong W, Kim AS, Huang IA, Farahany NA, Josephson SA. Inability to consent does not diminish the desirability of stroke thrombolysis. *Ann Neurol* 2014;76:296–304.
9. Clarke JL, Johnston SC, Farrant M, et al. External validation of the ICH score. *Neurocrit Care* 2004;1:53–60.
10. Desai JA, Smith EE. Prenotification and other factors involved in rapid tPA administration. *Curr Atheroscler Rep* 2013;15:337.
11. Edlow JA, Selim MH. Atypical presentations of acute cerebrovascular syndromes. *Lancet Neurol* 2011;10:550–560.
12. Evenson KR, Foraker RE, Morris DL, Rosamond WD. A comprehensive review of prehospital and in-hospital delay times in acute stroke care. *Int J Stroke* 2009;4:187–199.
13. Fawole A, Daw HA, Crowther MA. Practical management of bleeding due to the anticoagulants dabigatran, rivaroxaban, and apixaban. *Cleve Clin J Med* 2013;80:443–451.

14. Furlan AJ. Endovascular therapy for stroke—it's about time. *N Engl J Med* 2015 published on time.
15. Hemphill JC, 3rd, Bonovich DC, Besmertis L, Manley GT, Johnston SC. The ICH score: a simple, reliable grading scale for intracerebral hemorrhage. *Stroke* 2001;32:891–897.
16. Hickey M, Gatien M, Taljaard M, et al. Outcomes of urgent warfarin reversal with frozen plasma versus prothrombin complex concentrate in the emergency department. *Circulation* 2013;128:360–364.
17. Hill MD, Coutts SB. Alteplase in acute ischemic stroke: the need for speed. *Lancet* 2014;384:1904–1906.
18. Huang X, Cheripelli B, Lloyd SM. Alteplase versus tenecteplase for thrombolysis after ischemic stroke (ATTEST): a phase 2, randomized, open-label, blinded endpoint study. *Lancet Neurol* 2015;14:368–376.
19. Khosravani H, Mayer SA, Demchuk A, et al. Emergency noninvasive angiography for acute intracerebral hemorrhage. *AJNR Am J Neuroradiol* 2013;34:1481–1487.
20. Kostopoulos P, Walter S, Haass A, et al. Mobile stroke unit for diagnosis-based triage of persons with suspected stroke. *Neurology* 2012;78:1849–1852.
21. LaMonte MP, Cullen J, Gagliano DM, et al. TeleBAT: mobile telemedicine for the Brain Attack Team. *J Stroke Cerebrovasc Dis* 2000;9:128–135.
22. LaMonte MP, Xiao Y, Hu PF, et al. Shortening time to stroke treatment using ambulance telemedicine: TeleBAT. *J Stroke Cerebrovasc Dis* 2004;13:148–154.
23. Liman TG, Winter B, Waldschmidt C, et al. Telestroke ambulances in prehospital stroke management: concept and pilot feasibility study. *Stroke* 2012;43:2086–2090.
24. Meretoja A, Weir L, Ugalde M, et al. Helsinki model cut stroke thrombolysis delays to 25 minutes in Melbourne in only 4 months. *Neurology* 2013;81:1071–1076.
25. Naidech AM, Liebling SM, Rosenberg NF, et al. Early platelet transfusion improves platelet activity and may improve outcomes after intracerebral hemorrhage. *Neurocrit Care* 2012;16:82–87.
26. Prabhakaran S, O'Neill K, Stein-Spencer L, Walter J, Alberts MJ. Prehospital triage to primary stroke centers and rate of stroke thrombolysis. *JAMA Neurol* 2013;70:1126–1132.
27. Prabhakaran S, Silver AJ, Warrior L, McClenathan B, Lee VH. Misdiagnosis of transient ischemic attacks in the emergency room. *Cerebrovasc Dis* 2008;26:630–635.
28. Saver JL. Time is brain—quantified. *Stroke* 2006;37:263–266.
29. Scott PA, Xu Z, Meurer WJ, et al. Attitudes and beliefs of Michigan emergency physicians toward tissue plasminogen activator use in stroke: baseline survey results from the INcreasing Stroke Treatment through INteractive behavioral Change Tactic (INSTINCT) trial hospitals. *Stroke* 2010;41:2026–2032.
30. Steiner T, Al-Shahi Salman R, Beer R, et al. European Stroke Organisation (ESO) guidelines for the management of spontaneous intracerebral hemorrhage. *Int J Stroke* 2014;9:840–855.
31. Toyoda K, Steiner T, Epple C, et al. Comparison of the European and Japanese guidelines for the acute management of intracerebral hemorrhage. *Cerebrovasc Dis* 2013;35:419–429.
32. Van Hooff RJ, Cambron M, Van Dyck R, et al. Prehospital unassisted assessment of stroke severity using telemedicine: a feasibility study. *Stroke* 2013;44:2907–2909.
33. Van Hooff RJ, De Smedt A, De Raedt S, et al. Unassisted assessment of stroke severity using telemedicine. *Stroke* 2013;44:1249–1255.
34. Wijdicks EFM, Seth K, Carter B, et al. Recommendations for the management of cerebral and cerebellar infarction with swelling. *Stroke* 2014;45:1222–1238.

9

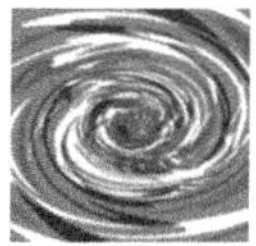

Triaging Acute Neuroinfections

While differences of presentation may be considerable, the main problem here is the broad differential diagnosis in a febrile confused patient. Many systemic illnesses produce fever and confusion, and in fact most of them do not involve the CNS. Missing a treatable acute CNS infection remains one of the most worrisome situations in acute neurology and perhaps in medicine as a whole. Repeatedly, in patients presenting with fever and confusion, acute bacterial meningitis, spinal abscess, or intracranial abscess is not considered. Thus, timely and prompt administration of IV antibiotics is delayed in a these patients despite cues pointing in that direction. Patients presenting with a new encephalitis may also be treated relatively late because presenting symptoms are nonspecific—sometimes only fluctuating orientation until stupor occurs. Herpes simplex encephalitis, may present with days of agitation and confusion until aphasia is diagnosed or focal seizures emerge.

Source identification remains one of the most important first considerations in febrile and sick patients. Important questions are as follows: How can we best identify CNS infections even if clinical signs and laboratory signs point toward another explanation? What is the best sequence of action in evaluating this patient? How can we initially and rapidly best treat these infections? What are the most common causes of encephalitis in the ED?

All of these topics are discussed in this chapter, which focuses on the major CNS infections. These are meningitis, brain or spinal abscesses. Encephalitis comes in seasonal waves but is seen by emergency physicians frequently enough to cause triage questions. More recently, it has become known that many encephalitides may have an autoimmune origin (management of these disorders is discussed in detail in *Handling Difficult Situations*). This chapter concentrates on neuroemergencies associated with bacterial CNS infections and viral encephalitis.

Principles

A few words need to be said about the pathophysiology of major CNS infections. First, bacterial meningitis commonly extends into the brain parenchyma and may also involve ventricles. In many cases, bacteremia precedes meningitis—the source might be choroid plexus, where bacteria may cross the blood–brain barrier and invade. Similar findings occur with epidural abscesses, where most likely there has been hematological spread. Most spinal cord infections are related to pyogenic spondylodiscitis, which may be a source of epidural abscesses. Therapeutic spinal injections are notorious for causing *Staphylococcus aureus* infections that may spread throughout the body, causing endocarditis and possibly an epidural abscess. Other causes for an epidural abscess are acutely infected surgical wounds or decubital ulcers.

The pathophysiology of any infection in the CNS is determined by survival of pathogens in the CSF and several steps that would allow the bacteria to cross the blood–brain barrier. Bacteria can spread through blood—which in children is predominantly seen coming from the nasopharynx—from a focal infection due to mastoiditis, or via a CSF leak with prior surgery or trauma. Cerebrospinal spinal fluid has several anti-inflammatory factors that suppress immune reactivity and bacteria multiply easily in the CSF. Virulence required for pathogenicity remains an important defining characteristic, and there are different mechanisms operating at the transcriptional and translational levels. Typically, a major inflammatory response leads to further bacterial invasion and leukocyte entry. This selectively activates production of cytokines and chemokines, resulting in recruitment of large amounts of neutrophils, in turn producing chemotactic agents that incite inflammation. This response eventually leads to vascular injury, vasogenic brain edema, increased ICP, and brain compression. Vasculitis can also produce cerebral infarcts, which can produce a mass effect, but most of the time smaller infarcts are seen. Other antimicrobial factors that are released into the extracellular space are matrix metalloproteinases, which is related to further breach of the blood–brain barrier. Because of this multiple pathophysiological cascade, several treatments can be devised that could reduce the inflammatory response while killing the bacteria with antibiotics.

The major pyogenic infections are meningitis, brain abscesses, and subdural empyema. Brain abscesses in general are located at the junction of the white matter and gray matter or in the territory of the lentiform arteries. Multiple abscesses have typically been associated seen with valvular heart disease or the presence of a pulmonary arteriovenous fistula, as in Rendu–Osler–Weber disease. Most of the time sources come from continuity due to an infection in the ear, sinus, or petrous bone. Hematogenic causes of brain abscesses are less common. In more than 10% of the cases, the cause of a brain abscess remains unresolved.

Rather than using CSF examination alone to prove infection, it may be more diagnostic to identify the damage to CNS structures with neuroimaging. Imaging of a pyrogenic infection is best done using MRI and in meningitis will show enhanced meninges and areas of cerebritis or infarction. Typically, MRI scan in an abscess shows a hyperintensity on T2-weighted images (in the cerebritis stage) and is hyperintense relative to CSF and hypodense relative to the white matter. Vasogenic edema is characterized by hypodensity on T1 images. A bright signal on a diffusion-weighted sequence and reduced apparent diffusion coefficient value is characteristic of a brain abscess but is not pathognomonic. MRI is the preferred

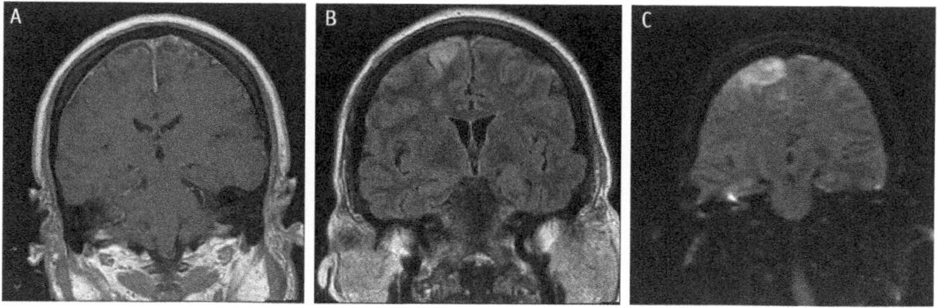

Figure 9.1 MRI of bacterial meningitis.

diagnostic test in epidural abcesses and can show one or more localizations. Examples are shown in Figures 9.1–9.3.

The pathophysiologic mechanisms of viral encephalitis are different, involving different CNS structures. The virus enters the CNS through hematogenic spread. Mosquitoes are often the vector. There is selective cellular vulnerability in the CNS; in some encephalitides (e.g., mumps), meninges are more affected, in others the anterior horn cells of the spinal cord are preferentially involved (West Nile virus and poliovirus). In brainstem encephalitis (Bickerstaff's encephalitis), there is edema and lymphocytic cuffing but no neuronal necrosis. Herpes simplex encephalitis is associated with hemorrhagic necrosis, specifically involving the temporal lobes, insula, and the posterior orbitofrontal cortex. The findings on neuropathology in encephalitis are generally nonspecific, showing clusters of inflammatory changes and, in some areas, perivascular chronic inflammation with microglial nodules and neuronophagia. When examined ultrastructurally, viral particles with hexagonal features and a

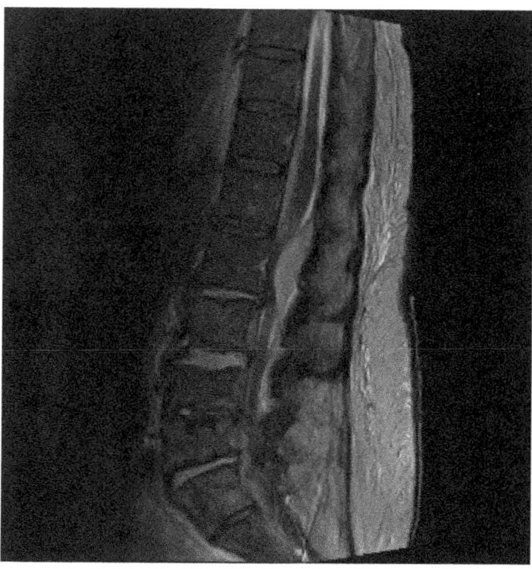

Figure 9.2 MRI of epidural abscess.

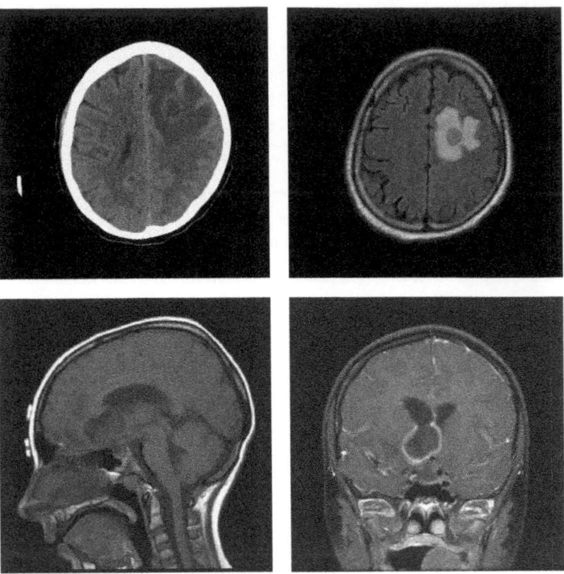

Figure 9.3 CT and MRI of cerebral abscess (upper row single abscess, lower row ventricular rupture of abscess).

central nucleoid can be found. Deep sequencing technologies on brain biopsy specimens can be helpful in finding the cause of viral encephalitis.

In Practice

There are several important steps to be considered that would facilitate recognition of CNS infections. Each of these infections and their potential pitfalls are discussed here.

BACTERIAL MENINGITIS

Meningitis remains a rare diagnosis, but one recent study identified 62 per 100,000 ED visits.[26] How is a bacterial meningitis recognized? In general, the presentation is a decreased level of consciousness—fully alert patients are likely not in the throes of a bacterial meningitis. A history of several days of excruciating headache is a useful clue. Nuchal rigidity and positive Brudzinski's sign (flexion in hips triggered by flexion in the neck) and Kernig's sign (passive extension of the knees with hips flexed) can be found, indicating meningeal inflammation. Some have argued that jolt accentuation (worsening headache with horizontal rotation of the neck two to three times per second) is an important indicator of meningitis. All these tests have a low sensitivity: jolt accentuation 21%, Kernig's sign 2%, Brudzinski's sign 2%, and nuchal rigidity 13%.[19]

Bacterial meningitis is often not recognized in a timely fashion.[2,12,28,30,31] Moreover, expertise of care may only be found in tertiary centers, implying that patients need quick transfer. When general hospitals are audited, the time from presentation to recognition of meningitis and time to initiation of diagnostic tests are markedly delayed. A recent study showed that the average time from entry to the ED to performance of CT scanning was on average 2½ hours and the time of diagnosis of meningitis to start of antibiotics was over 2 hours from entry.[24] The time to lumbar puncture was on average nearly 5 hours. Only 64% of the patients with suspected meningitis were treated with antibiotics before CT scan and lumbar puncture.[24] These findings are worrisom, but these delays may occur everywhere, indicating a more widespread problem.

The traditional line of action in any patient suspected of bacterial meningitis is to

- secure airway and stabilize blood pressure,
- treat seizures and IV load with levetiracetam,
- immediately obtain blood cultures,
- provide broad-spectrum IV antibiotics and corticosteroids,
- proceed with CT scan, and
- perform lumbar puncture if there is no coagulopathy.

Any deviation from this step by step approach could lead to failure to identify the microorganism or complications of interventions. For example, a lumbar puncture performed before a CT scan could lead to worsening of the patient if the cause is not bacterial meningitis but rather an epidural abscess with mass effect.

Four tubes of CSF are collected and investigated for red blood cells, white blood cells, protein, and glucose. One tube is specifically used for Gram stain and cultures. In some circumstances, polymerase chain reaction (PCR) for microbacteria is required. It is important to measure the spinal fluid pressure—elevation is defined as more than 200 mm H_2O. In meningitis, an abnormal CSF typically shows protein that is elevated and more than 50 mg/dL, a positive Gram stain, and an increased white blood cell count (usually more than 1,000 cells per μL).

Bacterial meningitis may present in a fulminant way, but this is not specifically related to the pathogen and it may be more attributable to drug resistance. Multiple drug resistant gram-negative bacilli have emerged in patients with healthcare-associated bacterial meningitis. It has been clearly established that a good outcome after bacterial meningitis can be achieved when patients are treated with rapid administration of appropriate antibiotics and corticosteroids if there are no major secondary complications such as brain edema on CT scan. However, one study found hydrocephalus in 50% of patients with fulminant bacterial meningitis and cerebral edema in 92%.[18] Poor outcome in fulminant bacterial meningitis can not only be related to less aggressive ICP management or sepsis but also to time to initiate antibiotics and dexamethasone in the ED. This procrastination was seen clearly in a recent study in France, where the average time from entry to treatment with antibiotics in the ED was 3 hours (1–5 hours range) and the time from entry to treatment with dexamethasone was 6 hours (2–9 hours).[17] The study reported an unfavorable outcome in patients who developed severe sepsis. Therefore, delay to diagnosis; delay to antibiotic treatment; delay to treatment of critical illness, especially sepsis and airway management; and delay of treatment of increased ICP remain major concerns in the management of acute bacterial meningitis. Mortality remains high in

Table 9.1 **Further Action Plan in a Patient with a Strong Suspicion of Bacterial Meningitis**

- CSF formula is diagnostic when
  - Glucose <34 mg/dL
  - CSF to serum glucose ratio <0.23
  - Protein >220 mg/dL
  - Total pleocytosis >2,000 cells/μL
  - Polymorphonuclear >1,180 cells/μL
- Cefotaxime 2 g IV (then every 12 hours)
- Vancomycin 20 mg/kg IV (then adjust and every 12 hours)
- Ampicillin 2 g IV (then every 6 hours)
- Dexamethasone 10 mg IV (then every 6 hours and for 10 days)
- Ventriculostomy with acute hydrocephalus
- Mannitol 1–2 g/kg with acute brain edema
- Obtain MRI if patient is not improving

CSF = cerebrospinal fluid; CT - computed tomography; MRI = magnetic resonance imaging.

fulminant bacterial meningitis (40%–50%, and in some studies 70%). Outcome is particularly poor in patients who have had splenectomy or have a hyposplenic state, and one study found unfavorable outcome in 58% and mortality in 25%.[1]

Finally, it is important to realize that bacterial meningitis may be part of a more systemic infection—endocarditis may be the primary culprit in patients with bacterial meningitis. This is a rare occurrence, but bacterial meningitis should be considered in patients who have *S. aureus*. In these patients, an echocardiogram should be performed immediately, after which appropriate further action should be undertaken after consultation with a cardiac surgeon

Streptococcus pneumoniae (or pneumococcus) is the most common cause of bacterial meningitis in adults. CSF Gram stain and cultures—but also blood cultures—readily and rapidly identify the bacteria in most cases. Infection with *Listeria monocytogenes* must be considered in elderly patients (over 60 years) and alcoholics, and can be adequately treated by adding ampicillin (or ciprofloxacin) to an already broad empiric regimen with vancomycin and a third-generation cephalosporin. A guideline for emergent intervention is shown in Table 9.1. Common organisms are shown in Table 9.2.

EPIDURAL SPINAL ABSCESS

An epidural spinal abscess is another emergency that is often not clearly recognized despite the fact that most patients present with paraparesis. Fifty percent of patients with spinal epidural abscesses are misdiagnosed at

Table 9.2 **Common Organisms in Bacterial Meningitis**

Organism	*Age*	*Risk Factors*	*Proportion of Cases*	*Case Fatality*
Streptococcus pneumoniae	All ages	Complement deficiency, asplenia, alcoholism	57%	18%; (doubles in immunocompromised patients)
Neisseria meningitidis	Age 11–17 years and younger adults	Multiperson dwellings, travel	17%	10%
Listeria monocytogenes	Neonates and adults	Cell-mediated immunodeficiencies (e.g., steroids, HIV, alcoholism), newborns	4%	18%
Haemophilus influenzae	Children and adults	Newborns	6%	7%
Group B streptococcus	Neonates	Often <2 months	17%	11%
Gram-negative rods (e.g., Escherichia coli, Klebsiella)	Adults	Nosocomial infection	33%	35% nosocomial; 25% community acquired

Source: Adapted from Bartt.[2]

presentation.[4,5,10,13,14,21–23] The cooperation of the otherwise sick patient to test muscle strength may play a role, but failing to do a sensory examination, failing to test anal muscle strength, or failure to obtain appropriate imaging studies is common impediments to recognition of spinal epidural abscesses. An epidural abscess should be considered if the patient presents with back pain and unexplained fever, if there have been prior injections (particularly epidural injections), recent spinal surgery, or if there is a predisposition for infections, as in patients with diabetes mellitus or IV drug use. About 20% of spinal lesions are associated with vertebral osteomyelitis, and therefore a plain spine X-ray may point toward that direction. An MRI is indispensible (CT scan of the spine is an insensitive test for an epidural abscess) (Figure 9.2). Patients with an epidural abscess may have significant neck pain, which may look like meningitis. Neurologic examination should identify level of disease, the presence of bowel and bladder dysfunction, and possibly osteomyelitis, which requires consultation with spine surgeons. Recognition of weakness, usually in the lower extremities due to the predominance of epidural abscesses in the thoracolumbar area, is important, as this requires immediate neurosurgical intervention and drainage of the abscess and long-term IV antibiotics.

Surgical intervention is only possible if the abscess can be drained in a localized area. Medical management typically fails in patients who have significant leukocytosis, underlying diabetes mellitus, positive blood cultures, and a C-reactive protein greater than 5 mg/dl and often 10-15 mg/dl.[20] Medical management leads to some improvement in about 1 in 10 patients.

A spinal cord epidural abscess above the conus has a different outcome simply because small abscesses may not necessarily cause clinical symptoms other than an infection. Four major factors increase the probability of failure: age more than 65 years old, diabetes, methicillin-resistant *S. aureus* (MRSA), and neurological impairment. In patients older than 65 years with no other risk factors—no diabetes, no MRSA, and no neurologic impairment—there is still a 33% risk of treatment failure. This rapidly increases to 50%–60% with two risk factors present. With all four risk factors present, there is a 99% chance of treatment failure.[15]

A recent study found that evacuation within 24 hours may not significantly benefit patients, but there were important trends suggesting early intervention is worthwhile. Patients in the delayed surgery group were nearly a decade older, which may have biased the surgeon and thus the result.[10] A treatment guide is shown in Table 9.3.

BRAIN ABSCESS

Brain abscesses are unusual and often not suspected. Many patients have CT scan abnormalities that show vague hypodensities alone. Some of these CT scans are misread as new ischemic strokes, but contrast administration very often shows a ring-like lesion. The radiologic challenge is to differentiate between abscess and glioma, and both MRI and SPECT (single photon emission computed tomography) are helpful in making that distinction. Diffusion-weighted imaging shows an abnormal signal in abscess (not in tumor), but in immunosuppressed patients, disorders such as progressive multifocal leukoencephalopathy or lymphoma may show similar image characteristics.[8] Many patients present with headache alone. Nausea, fever, and decreased level of consciousness is not common—at least initially. Predisposing conditions are present in most patients; therefore, an ED evaluation by an otorhinolaryngologist, cardiologist or dentist might be indicated to find the source of the infection in ear, sinus, heart valve or root canal.

Table 9.3 **Action Plan with Strong Suspicion of Epidural Abscess**

- Start vancomycin 20 mg/kg/day in divided doses every 12 hours
- Start metronidazole 500 mg (continue every 6 hours)
- Start cefotaxime 2 g (continuing every 4 hours)
- Urgent neurosurgeon consult for laminectomy and drainage if single mass

Table 9.4 **Action Plan with Strong Suspicion of Cerebral Abscess**

- Start cefotaxime 2 g (continue every 4 hours)
- Start metronidazole 500 mg (continue every 6 hours) or meropenem 2 g (continue every 8 hours)
- Start vancomycin 20 mg/kg (continue every 12 hours)
- Start voriconazole 4 mg/kg (continue every 12 hours)
- Consider tuberculosis triple therapy if likely (Isoniazid, rifampin, pyrazinamide, ethambutol)
- Contact neurosurgeon and obtain MRI with fiducials

MRI = magnetic resonance imaging.

Generally, the neurosurgical approach to a brain abscess is stereotactic aspiration and drainage or, if closer to the surface, excision. Aspiration is less likely to cause additional neurologic deficits when compared with excision and often can be done with a simple burr hole. Most reports emphasize a good outcome with 70%–80% of the patients, although focal deficits remain and postoperative seizures are a continuous concern. Antiepileptic drugs should be started almost immediately. An urgent situation arises in patients who have an intraventricular rupture of the abscess (Figure 9.3). These patients require evacuation with lavage of the ventricles and ventriculostomy placement, followed by intraventricular antibiotics. Cerebellar abscess is another neurosurgical emergency and treatment involves excision of the abscess to reduce brainstem compression. Most of these patients have cerebellar abscesses in the setting of mastoiditis, and an ENT consultation is necessary for simultaneous surgery. Multiple abscesses would require antibiotic treatment, and in general, only abscesses more than 2.5 cm in size are drained. Treatment for cerebral abscess should include vancomycin, cefepime, and metronidazole. Meropenem is not a good choice because of its seizure proclivity.[3] IV antibiotics may also include intraventricular administration of gentamicin twice daily for 6 weeks. A guideline is shown in Table 9.4.

VIRAL ENCEPHALITIS

Viral infection is the most common cause of acute encephalitis in adults.[25,26] Encephalitis comes in seasons, usually in the summer. Large numbers of patients often point to a possible cause (e.g., Japanese encephalitis).[7] Epidemic outbreaks can be produced by the seasonal spread of arboviruses (i.e. viruses transmitted by arthropod vectors, such as mosquitoes). Most of these agents are constrained to specific geographical locations, but there are exceptions such as the West Nile virus, which has been identified as a cause of summer outbreaks of encephalitis in all continents. Viral encephalitis is mostly sporadic and occur in the immunocompetent and the immunocompromised. In the United States, over the last decade, over 200,000 cases of encephalitis were diagnosed; the total numbers have been stable when compared with the prior decade. HIV-associated encephalitides, particularly *Toxoplasma* encephalitis, declined.[32] Viral causes of encephalitis are found in nearly 50% of cases.[9] Mortality is highest in the elderly and in patients with HIV/AIDS and other medical illness. Encephalitis associated with transplantation may have increased. In the weeks after transplantation, reactivation of a CNS viral infection is mostly seen in bone marrow transplant recipients, often involving herpes viruses such as herpes simplex virus type 1 (HSV-1), varicella-zoster virus, and the most notorious human herpes virus 6. *Mycobacterium tuberculosis* was frequent cause of encephalitis in one study from France.[25]

Autoimmune encephalitis (typically in young and previously healthy females) is more commonly recognized and has a much better outcome as a result of immunotherapy (see the volume *Handling Difficult Situations*).

Patients with a viral encephalitis present with headache, fever, confusion, and, when the encephalitis is more advanced, abnormal consciousness. Examination may show neck stiffness or focal deficits, but there may be no localizing signs. Seizures or nonconvulsive status epilepticus may occur. While the CT scan can be highly suggestive of certain forms of encephalitis, radiological changes are generally not characteristic of specific encephalitis etiologies. A brain MRI is far more helpful. CSF showing increased white blood cell count and an increased protein concentration confirms the presence of encephalitis. A normal CSF strongly argues for considering alternative diagnoses (such as noninfectious limbic encephalitis). PCR of CSF is better in identifying DNA viruses (e.g., HSV) than RNA viruses (e.g., West Nile virus).[6,11,16,25,27,29,32,33]

The most frequent cause of sporadic viral encephalitis in immunocompetent patients is HSV-1 encephalitis, which has a predilection for the temporal lobes, insula, and operculum. Consequently, this should be suspected when febrile patients develop confusion seizures or focal deficits referable to those locations. Aphasia, amnesia, hallucinations, and agitation can be seen.

When encephalitis is present, the typical distribution of early swelling on brain MRI strongly supports the diagnosis. Nonetheless, the diagnosis should be established by confirming the presence of the virus in the CSF. PCR can detect HSV-1 DNA in the CSF with great sensitivity and specificity. If PCR is negative but the clinical and radiological presentation is suspicious for HSV-1 infection, the test should be repeated on a new CSF sample after 3–5 days.

EEG should be performed in patients with HSV-1 encephalitis. It is not unusual to see patients with encephalitis who exhibit fluctuating levels of alertness and awareness. In these cases, we often pursue continuous EEG monitoring, particularly in comatose patients with encephalitis. Nonconvulsive seizures are not uncommon but EEG patterns should be differentiated from periodic lateralized epileptiform discharges.

All patients with presumed acute encephalitis should be started immediately on IV acyclovir (10 mg/kg every 8 hours with longer intervals between doses in case of reduced glomerular filtration rate). This antiviral agent is the first choice for treating HSV-1, HSV-2, and varicella-zoster virus. Cytomegalovirus infection requires the combination of ganciclovir and foscarnet. Ganciclovir and foscarnet are also the treatment for HSV-6 infection in immunosuppressed patients. No antiviral has proven effective against West Nile virus infection. Patients coinfected with HIV must receive highly active antiretroviral therapy. In cases of progressive multifocal leukoencephalopathy (JC virus), the treatment consists of reversing immunosuppression (Table 9.5).

The management of acute encephalitis requires admission to an ICU. The major issues are recognition and treatment of seizures requiring video/EEG monitoring, and mechanical ventilation in patients unable to protect the airway. Patients who develop brain swelling might require ICP monitoring. Intraparenchymal monitors are preferable when the ventricles are compressed by brain edema. The most severe cases may demand decompressive craniectomy. Corticosteroids do not have a role in the treatment of viral encephalitis.

TRIAGE

All CNS infections require ICU admission and infectious disease consultant involvement. In bacterial meningitis antibiotics and corticosteroids must be administered in the ED. Appropriate neuroimaging is warranted emergently to triage more appropriately. Neurosurgery involvement is common in abscesses (to proceed with biopsy or ventriculostomy).

Table 9.5 **Main Causes of Acute Viral Encephalitis, Diagnostic Tests, and Principal Aspects of Management**

Causes	*Tests*	*Management Principles*
HSV-1	CSF PCR	Acyclovir, exclude seizures
VZV	CSF PCR	Acyclovir +/− corticosteroids
CMV	CSF PCR	Ganciclovir + foscarnet, exclude HIV
WNV	Serum IgM	Supportive
Influenza	Viral culture, antigen, and PCR of respiratory tract specimen	Oseltamivir
Other arboviruses	CSF serology	Supportive, exclude seizures
JC virus (PML)	CSF PCR	Reverse immunosuppression HAART if HIV
HIV	CSF PCR (viral load)	HAART
Measles	Serum and CSF Ab PCR of nasopharynx, urine, brain	Ribavirin if life-threatening
Mumps	Serum and CSF Ab	Supportive
Rabies	Serum and CSF Ab (if unvaccinated) IMF of viral antigen in nuchal skin biopsy Brain pathology	No treatment other than treatment for dysautonomia

HSV-1 = herpes simplex virus type 1; CSF = cerebrospinal fluid; PCR = polymerase chain reaction; CMV = cytomegalovirus; HIV = human immunodeficiency virus; WNV = West Nile virus; IgM = immunoglobulin M; PML = progressive multifocal leukoencephalopathy; HAART = highly active antiretroviral therapy; Ab = antibody; IMF = immunofluorescence.

Putting It All Together

- The treatment of meningitis requires step by step logical approach.
- Sepsis and meningitis is associated with much worse outcome.
- Epidural spinal abscess is not commonly recognized.
- Source finding in cerebral abscess is often unsuccessful.

By the Way

- Fulminant meningitis is associated with cerebral venous thrombosis.
- Fulminant meningitis often is associated with ventriculitis.
- Epidural abscess can present with bacteremia only.
- Intraventricular rupture of a cerebral abscess may worsen prognosis.

Triaging Acute Neuroinfections by the Numbers

- ~90% of patients have positive bacterial culture in CSF
- ~80% of patients have positive bacterial culture in serum
- ~70% of patients have a predisposing condition with brain abscess
- ~70% mortality in bacterial meningitis and sepsis
- ~20% mortality in bacterial meningitis when antibiotics administered early

References

1. Adriani KS, Brouwer MC, van der Ende A, van de Beek D. Bacterial meningitis in adults after splenectomy and hyposplenic states. *Mayo Clin Proc* 2013;88:571–578.
2. Bartt R. Acute bacterial and viral meningitis. *Continuum (Minneap Minn)* 2012;18:1255–1270.
3. Brouwer MC, Tunkel AR, McKhann GM, 2nd, van de Beek D. Brain abscess. *N Engl J Med* 2014;371:447–456.
4. Darouiche RO. Spinal epidural abscess. *N Engl J Med* 2006;355:2012–2020.
5. Davis DP, Wold RM, Patel RJ, et al. The clinical presentation and impact of diagnostic delays on emergency department patients with spinal epidural abscess. *J Emerg Med* 2004;26:285–291.
6. Emig M, Apple DJ. Severe West Nile virus disease in healthy adults. *Clin Infect Dis* 2004;38:289–292.
7. Feng Y, Fu S, Zhang H, et al. High incidence of Japanese encephalitis, southern China. *Emerg Infect Dis* 2013;19:672–673.
8. Finelli PF, Foxman EB. The etiology of ring lesions on diffusion-weighted imaging. *Neuroradiol J* 2014;27:280–287.
9. George BP, Schneider EB, Venkatesan A. Encephalitis hospitalization rates and inpatient mortality in the United States, 2000–2010. *PLoS One* 2014;9:e104169.
10. Ghobrial GM, Beygi S, Viereck MJ, et al. Timing in the surgical evacuation of spinal epidural abscesses. *Neurosurg Focus* 2014;37:E1.

11. Glaser CA, Honarmand S, Anderson LJ, et al. Beyond viruses: clinical profiles and etiologies associated with encephalitis. *Clin Infect Dis* 2006;43:1565–1577.
12. Heckenberg SG, de Gans J, Brouwer MC, et al. Clinical features, outcome, and meningococcal genotype in 258 adults with meningococcal meningitis: a prospective cohort study. *Medicine* 2008;87:185–192.
13. Huang PY, Chen SF, Chang WN, et al. Spinal epidural abscess in adults caused by *Staphylococcus aureus*: clinical characteristics and prognostic factors. *Clin Neurol Neurosurg* 2012;114:572–576.
14. Karikari IO, Powers CJ, Reynolds RM, Mehta AI, Isaacs RE. Management of a spontaneous spinal epidural abscess: a single-center 10-year experience. *Neurosurgery* 2009;65:919–923; discussion 923–914.
15. Kim SD, Melikian R, Ju KL, et al. Independent predictors of failure of nonoperative management of spinal epidural abscesses. *Spine J* 2015;15:95–101.
16. McGrath N, Anderson NE, Croxson MC, Powell KF. Herpes simplex encephalitis treated with acyclovir: diagnosis and long term outcome. *J Neurol Neurosurg Psychiatry* 1997;63:321–326.
17. Mourvillier B, Tubach F, van de Beek D, et al. Induced hypothermia in severe bacterial meningitis: a randomized clinical trial. *JAMA* 2013;310:2174–2183.
18. Muralidharan R, Mateen FJ, Rabinstein AA. Outcome of fulminant bacterial meningitis in adult patients. *Eur J Neurol* 2014;21:447–453.
19. Nakao JH, Jafri FN, Shah K, Newman DH. Jolt accentuation of headache and other clinical signs: poor predictors of meningitis in adults. *Am J Emerg Med* 2014;32:24–28.
20. Patel AR, Alton TB, Bransford RJ, et al. Spinal epidural abscesses: risk factors, medical versus surgical management, a retrospective review of 128 cases. *Spine J* 2014;14:326–330.
21. Rigamonti D, Liem L, Sampath P, et al. Spinal epidural abscess: contemporary trends in etiology, evaluation, and management. *Surg Neurol* 1999;52:189–196.
22. Rigamonti D, Metellus P. Spinal epidural abscess. *N Engl J Med* 2007;356:638.
23. Sampath P, Rigamonti D. Spinal epidural abscess: a review of epidemiology, diagnosis, and treatment. *J Spinal Disord* 1999;12:89–93.
24. Schuh S, Lindner G, Exadaktylos AK, Muhlemann K, Tauber MG. Determinants of timely management of acute bacterial meningitis in the ED. *Am J Emerg Med* 2013;31:1056–1061.
25. Sonneville R, Gault N, de Montmollin E, et al. Clinical spectrum and outcomes of patients with encephalitis requiring intensive care. *Eur J Neurol* 2015;22:6–16.
26. Takhar SS, Ting SA, Camargo CA, Jr., Pallin DJ. U.S. emergency department visits for meningitis, 1993–2008. *Acad Emerg Med* 2012;19:632–639.
27. Thakur KT, Motta M, Asemota AO, et al. Predictors of outcome in acute encephalitis. *Neurology* 2013;81:793–800.
28. Thigpen MC, Whitney CG, Messonnier NE, et al. Bacterial meningitis in the United States, 1998–2007. *N Engl J Med* 2011;364:2016–2025.
29. Tyler KL, Pape J, Goody RJ, Corkill M, Kleinschmidt-DeMasters BK. CSF findings in 250 patients with serologically confirmed West Nile virus meningitis and encephalitis. *Neurology* 2006;66:361–365.
30. van de Beek D, de Gans J, Spanjaard L, et al. Clinical features and prognostic factors in adults with bacterial meningitis. *N Engl J Med* 2004;351:1849–1859.
31. van de Beek D, de Gans J, Tunkel AR, Wijdicks EF. Community-acquired bacterial meningitis in adults. *N Engl J Med* 2006;354:44–53.
32. Vora NM, Holman RC, Mehal JM, et al. Burden of encephalitis-associated hospitalizations in the United States, 1998–2010. *Neurology* 2014;82:443–451.
33. Whitley RJ. Herpes simplex encephalitis: adolescents and adults. *Antiviral Res* 2006;71:141–148.

10

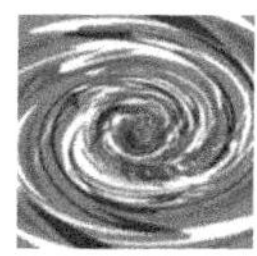

Troubleshooting: Errors and Misjudgments

Avoiding errors is the focus of quality improvement programs in the ED. In the ED patients present anew and over again and that is always a challenge. This also applies to the field of acute neurology. Neurologists or residents who are meticulous and organized on the ward may feel completely insecure and lose their footing in the ED. There is high demand ("cannot do all at once"), high action ("something has to be done now to stabilize the patient"), high risk ("the patient is worsening in front of my eyes"), and high stress ("am I correct here?") and, most of all, you are on your own ("I cannot get my consultant to answer his page"). Errors imprint in memory and never go away. There is a potential for improvement in any hospital situation, but medical errors and clinical risk management with patient contact in the ED are among the priorities being considered by administrators.[6] Rhetoric aside, some have argued that the number of errors is large and that what we are seeing is only a tip-of-the-iceberg phenomenon. Errors have been related to duty hours and overcrowding, but most errors have simple origins that involve diagnosis and treatment and potentially preventable situations. EDs are high-risk areas for medication errors, both prescription and administration. (Barcode technology has significantly reduced the frequency.[25,28,31]) In addition, and particularly in the ED, there is always a concern with incomplete information about the patient. Often the course of illness demands quick action and there is no room for leisurely gathering of information (Chapter 1). Some errors do harm the patient; others are inconsequential but must be recognized and prevented in the future. It can be argued that errors will become less common when expertise and knowledge are improved, but this is not always the case. Even a seasoned, highly active, and involved physician may get fooled or simply be unable to avoid an error because it presents anew. Much of what we do in medicine is pattern recognition, but the pattern must be known to avoid an error. This closing chapter provides some experiences and some reasoned explanation of where we can find the most common misjudgments. To understand errors, we have to understand how clinical decisions are made—good luck with that, many of us will say.

Basic Concepts of Clinical Judgment and Bias

Cognitive psychologists have provided insight into the bias that surrounds clinical judgment, offering a dual process model of thinking and reasoning that posits two main types of decision-makers.[18,24,32,34] Type I—most likely to cause error—uses thinking processes that are fast and intuitive. Type II is analytic, slow, and deliberate.[13,29] Type I may override type II (physicians going their own way), or type II may override type I (physician takes a diagnostic "time-out" and reflects). Type-I physicians may be molded by personality; type-II physicians are more likely acting as a result of rationality and critical thinking, asking themselves not only whether they are being comprehensive but also whether they have considered the most important cognitive biases.[11]

Some of the biases that surround clinical judgment has been identified and defined in Table 10.1. Knowledge of these potential problems is definitively interesting and may be helpful, but it is far from certain if it changes practice.[14]

Clinical experience does not reduce error rate—physicians often make the same mistake repeatedly. Diagnostic error in neurology is not exactly known, but where the whole of clinical medicine is concerned, some estimates have placed it at 15%.[10]

Table 10.1 **Cognitive Biases and Failed Heuristics**

Bias or Heuristic	*Definition/Display*
Anchoring	The tendency to lock on to salient features of the patient's presentation too early in the diagnostic process and failing to change this impression with later information.
Availability	The disposition to judge things as being more likely or frequently occurring, if they readily come to mind.
Base-rate neglect	The tendency to ignore the true prevalence of a disease, either inflating or reducing it.
Premature closure	The decision-making process ends too soon; the diagnosis is accepted before it has been fully verified.
Representativeness restraint	The physician looks for prototypical manifestations of disease (pattern recognition) and fails to consider atypical variants.
Search satisfying	The tendency to call off a search once something is found.
Unpacking principle	The failure to elicit all relevant information in establishing a differential diagnosis.
Context errors	The critical signal is distorted by the background against which it is perceived.

Source: Adapted from Croskerry et al.[5]

Errors are less frequent in specialties based on visual interpretation (~2%) and more frequent in clinical settings when there are multiple layers of interpretation.

Some have argued that overconfidence may play a role. Such an attitude may be reflected in failure to use resources, failure to consult colleagues, or simply failure to ask for help when it would be best for the patient. Moreover, clinical guidelines may be followed irregularly, which could reflect skepticism ("all low level of evidence and personal opinion") and also failure to diagnose the disorder to which the guideline applies. Many causes of errors can be categorized as premature diagnosis with no follow-up, premature tendency to seek out signs that fit the first impression, and a bias regarding the history. Complacency is the worst cause of error, caused by the general assumption that errors are inevitable and that in most situations another decision would not have affected outcome.[2] Others have suggested that, at the fellow or resident level, blind obedience to authority may be a major pitfall and such behavior or personal interaction can only change by fostering an environment with close communication, transparency, explanation, and mutual respect.[34]

Error Recognition

Errors can be divided into system errors and physician errors. System errors are errors in triage, teamwork, communication, and malfunction of equipment. Physician errors include diagnostic error (clinical, laboratory, and radiographic findings) or deviation from a usual procedure. Errors in medicine have been further defined in Table 10.2, and a deconstruction of events may be helpful in identifying a fix. Errors can be set apart from near misses (with some overlap) and from adverse events (Figure 10.1). An error could result from a collection of errors (misinterpretation of laboratory and examination), resulting in misdiagnosis or failure to come to a diagnosis. This may occur in about 30% of all neurologic diagnoses, though it may be higher in less serious neurologic diagnoses. High percentages of diagnostic error occur in brainstem or cerebellar stroke when the patient presents with vertigo, stroke or TIA, seizures, Guillain-Barré (GBS), myasthenia gravis, or spinal cord compression.[5,7,19,22,26,27,33]

One study found that 0.8% of 43,979 patients with Bell's palsy received an alternative diagnosis,[12] including stroke.[1] One in 10 patients with an alternative diagnosis

Table 10.2 **Types of Errors**

Violation	Failure to adhere to procedure or common practice
Procedural	Procedure followed but error during task
Communication	Error in exchange of information
Proficiency	Error due to lack of knowledge
Decision	Decisions increasing risk to patient

Source: Adapted from Helmreich.[16]

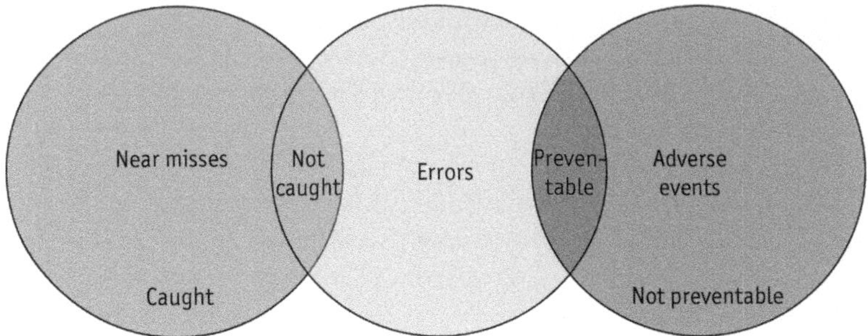

Figure 10.1 Errors, near misses, and adverse events.

had Guillain-Barré syndrome. (This is highly unusual considering that variants of GBS often present with other cranial nerves resulting in ophtalmoparesis or even more rarely present with bifacial palsy.)

Near misses may be caught in time and may involve failure to recognize acute hydrocephalus (CT scan points toward a reversible cause of coma) and failure to recognize meningitis (CSF finds abnormal formula requiring immediate antibiotics). A near miss may become an error if not caught in time; examples are medication errors (i.e., too low dosing of phenytoin in seizures). In some cases, a near miss that is not intercepted may have the potential for doing harm, but the patient is not harmed due to chance or some other characteristic of the patient. Medication errors may involve mathematical errors, usually with decimals. Electronic records could drastically reduce these errors.

Types of Errors in the Emergency Department

The types of errors by both neurologists and emergency physicians in the ED are shown in Table 10.3. They may involve diagnostic errors, and in acute neurology, there are multiple initial concerns. Most commonly, there is a failure to recognize the presence of an acute brain injury on a CT scan and failure to perform a CSF examination. This is clearly related to whether ED physicians have sufficient knowledge in the management of critically ill neurologic patients, and may be less in EDs where neurologists are present in a timely fashion (again arguing for camaraderie, hence this book). Failure to obtain an appropriate test such as an MRI scan in a patient with a spinal cord compression or failure to recognize the possibility of a neurointerventional option are errors that can potentially be avoided. Medication errors in the ED as a result of dose miscalculation, inappropriate route, or failure to adjust the dose in chronic kidney injury are less common. More common is delay in treatment initiation or a substandard approach regarding infectious disease.

Medical errors can be technical (e.g., misplacement of catheter, tube, or device; continuation of drug despite adverse drug reaction), judgmental (e.g., misdiagnosis of SAH, failure to recognize the rapidity and seriousness of spinal cord compression or mass effect and pending cerebral brain shift in a patient with a brain tumor), or normative (e.g., nondisclosure of risk, breach of confidentiality).

Table 10.3 **Types of Errors in the Emergency Department**

Diagnostic
• No conclusive diagnosis • Delay in diagnosis • Failure to obtain appropriate tests • Failure to act on test results
Treatment
• Wrong procedure or test • Wrong drug administered • Wrong dose (or failure to adjust dose) of drug • Delay in treatment initiation • "Substandard" approach
Preventive
• Inadequate follow-up of patient or triage • Lack of communication • Lack of planning

Common Slip-ups

Serious mistakes could occur in the ED and may cause permanent morbidity or premature death. Disclosure of mistakes may be deferred because of fear of a negligence suit or punitive responses by colleagues or simply failure to accept responsibility or blaming it all on someone else. An emergency physician missing a neurologic diagnosis may raise the question whether a neurologic assessment in that particular situation could have led to a diagnosis. Three studies have looked into the impact of neurology consultations on outcome of patients with neurologic emergencies. In France, neurology consults were obtained in approximately 50% of all patients and a change in diagnosis was found in over 50% of cases.[23] This study was flawed by providing additional test results to the neurologists, facilitating the diagnosis. In Canada, a study of 493 patients with neurologic emergencies found that in 60% of the cases the ED diagnosis remained unchanged. In the remaining cases, there was disagreement, or "significant uncertainty."[22] In a study of 500 neurology consultations in a tertiary academic hospital in the United States, nearly 5% of all ED patients had a neurologic consultation; it found prolonged length of stay among patients who had a neurologic consultation, more often in patients with diagnostic ambiguity.[15]

Several important categories of misdiagnosis have been identified. The first is misdiagnosis of a major neurologic disorder associated with headache. This includes SAH, which remains a challenging situation because in emergency room, populations in general less than 20% of patients with a classic thunderclap headache have an SAH.[3,8,9] Headache associated with cerebral venous thrombosis and dissections in the carotid or vertebral artery territory are commonly misdiagnosed. The second category is vertigo and dizziness, usually only rarely associated with an ischemic stroke.[21] It is unclear whether the neurologist is better than the emergency physician at diagnosing the important cause of dizziness.

The third important category is misdiagnosis of cauda equina syndrome in a patient with back pain. Here the problem may be an inability to perform an MRI scan in a patient with new back pain and insignificant weakness despite marked compression. Studies have found that new pain in elderly patients, prior cancer, fever, weight loss, immunocompromised state, IV drug use, recent urinary tract infection or bacteremia, pain worse at night, and the presence of sphincter syndromes and bilateral sciatica are important clues. Any patient with prior spinal procedure or injections or on anticoagulation requires an MRI scan if a new back pain occurs. Often, inadequate history, inadequate physical examination, or communication breakdown between physicians and nursing staff have been identified. In addition, less than 20% present with bilateral sciatica, leg weakness, saddle anesthesia, and sphincter dysfunction.[17] Another cause of weakness that is commonly misdiagnosed is GBS, particularly if patients present with paresthesia alone. It is understandable that rare disorders such as Lambert–Eaton syndrome and myasthenia gravis will lead to delay in diagnosis. A common problem (discussed in Chapter 4) is to distinguish syncope, epileptic seizures, and pseudoseizures. Syncopes usually have characteristic prodromes with a feeling of the world closing in, lightheadedness, sweating, and pallor noted by an observer. Often there is a precipitant. A cardiac cause of syncope may result in palpitations. When syncope is a result of epileptic seizure, tonic–clonic jerking is usually seen, including tongue biting and an abnormal blood gas suggesting metabolic acidosis often caused by increased lactate.

Illustrative Case Examples of Errors

In closing, a few cases may demonstrate how mistakes are made and, in particular, how easily this can occur.

CASE #1: FAILURE TO RECOGNIZE SERIOUSNESS

Description

A 62-year-old woman was seen in the ED with acute isolated vertigo. Her examination showed mild bilateral dysmetria and past-pointing. There was a barely noticeable dysarthria. The CT scan showed loss of gray–white differentiation in the inferior left cerebellar hemisphere. The patient was admitted to a stroke ward, but hours later became more drowsy. The CT scan (Figure 10.2) showed increased mass effect and obstructive hydrocephalus. Emergency suboccipital craniotomy was performed. She recovered well.

Comment

Cerebellar infarcts are notorious for rapid progression, while neurologic examination and CT are not diagnostic or are frankly misleading. If a suspicion exists,

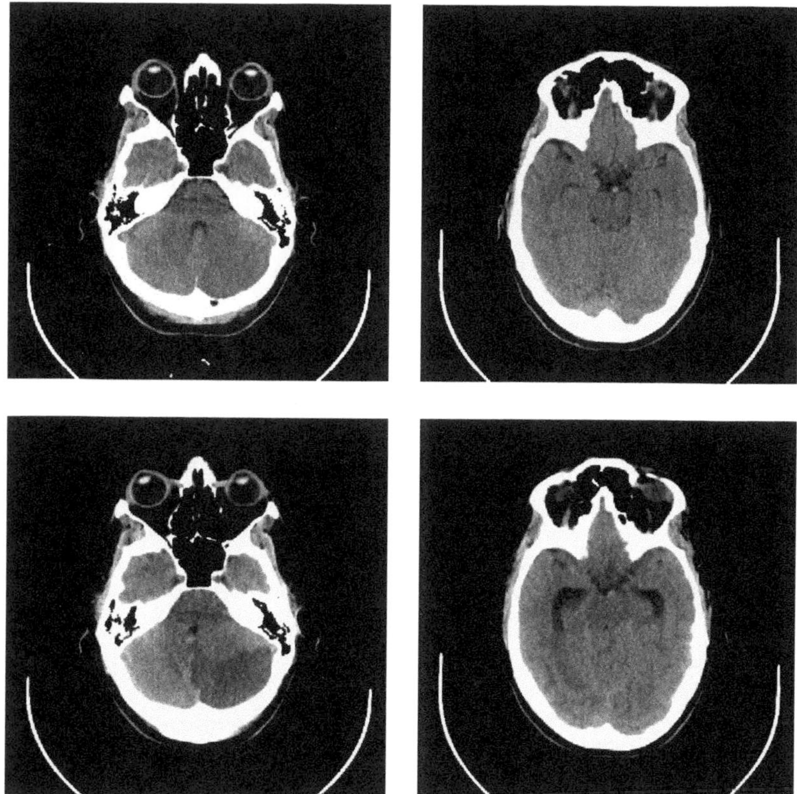

Figure 10.2 Developing mass effect and hydrocephalus after cerebellar infarct.

these patients require close monitoring in an ICU setting and a repeat CT scan 6–8 hours after admission. Some patients may suddenly develop apneic spells from brainstem compression, and neurosurgical evacuation is needed.

CASE #2: FAILURE TO ACT

Description

This is a 53-year-old woman who fell in the bathroom 10 days before being seen in the ED. Perhaps she lost consciousness, but she was not sure. She had developed headaches 3 days after the fall and gradually more nausea. Her speech was also more "hesitant" and "stuttering." Her neurologic examination was completely normal. The CT scan (Figure 10.3) revealed a small 1.5-cm thick subdural hematoma with mixed density indicating subacute and acute components. There was mass effect and a 1-cm midline shift. The right lateral ventricle was trapped. She was admitted to the ward, but the next day was found to have "new-onset" weakness. She remained alert but was "more" confused. She underwent neurosurgical evacuation and fully recovered.

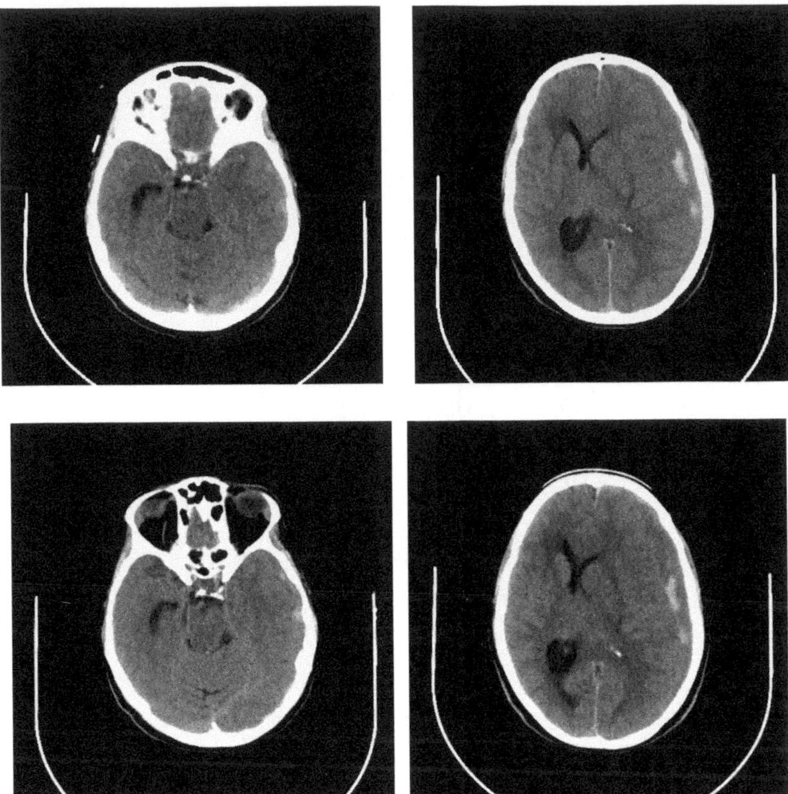

Figure 10.3 Worsening shift from subacute subdural hematoma.

Comment

A sizable subdural hematoma may worsen (or was worsening, with the patient developing nausea). The degree of shift would have warranted emergent neurosurgical consultation and may have led to evacuation urgently, or at least admission to a more secure environment. The fall several days ago and "normal" neurologic examination may have caused the error in judgment.

CASE # 3: FAILURE TO THINK OUTSIDE THE BOX

Description

A 63-year-old male was seen in the ED with a syncope. He had hit his head, but after a brief period of unconsciousness was lucid. This was followed by another syncope—he woke up on the sidewalk. On arrival, he was tachycardic and had a major frontal bruise. His CT scan was normal. His EKG showed a new right bundle branch block and mildly increased troponin. The neurologists felt that this finding was unusual for a mild head injury and consulted a cardiologist to look for a possible cardiac arrhythmia as an explanation for his syncope. An EKG showed severe right ventricular enlargement,

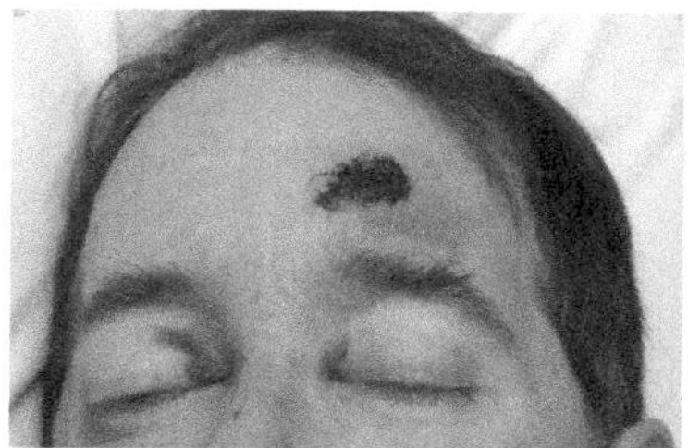 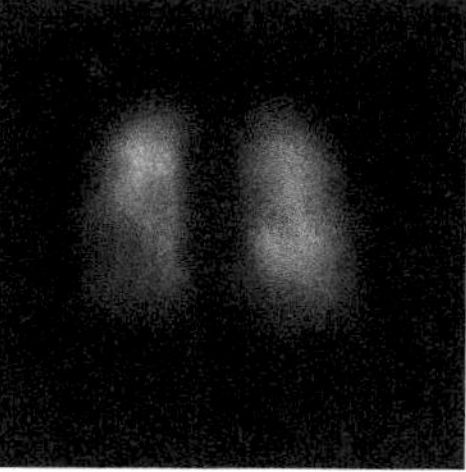

Figure 10.4 Local bruise from head injury after collapse. Perfusion scan shows pulmonary emboli as cause of syncope.

confirmed with echocardiography, and bilateral pulmonary emboli were subsequently diagnosed (Figure 10.4).

Comment

This example serves as a reminder to consider unusual causes of syncope and not concentrate on head injury alone. Visible head injury and syncope may seem a sufficient explanation for this event. EKG abnormalities did point toward an unusual cause, and even a transesophageal echocardiogram had to point to pulmonary emboli, finding a right ventricular strain. Physicians may fail to perceive important signs and try to force everything into a more recognizable scenario. Often it is useful to explain away incongruities, but sometime there is an important observation that requires explanation.

Error Management

Most errors happen because someone "did not know that" and "was not aware of that." Day-to-day errors are very common and not unique to acute neurology. Simulation centers could be used to train physicians in error avoidance. Recognition and discussion of potential specific errors in small-group discussion is an effective way to work against major defense mechanisms such as rejecting responsibility, emotional detachment, or—worse—feeling incompetent or unworthy. Not all bad things happen for a reason, but some do, and there might be a clear sequence of events that must be remedied. Downplaying errors does nobody good, nor does it improve confidence. Debriefing after an error and open discussion with family improves performance later.[20,30,35–38] Disciplinary actions for common errors are practically unnecessary. Physicians are best off being candid and having a sense of fairness and openness to outside concerns, and families will appreciate such a communication. Resisting and denying is poor decorum.

Motives for filing malpractice claims may involve perception of negligence, such as perceived treatment error or delay, missed or delayed diagnosis, equipment misuse, and pharmacologic mishaps. Injury may be difficult to prove because of the critical illness of the patient and the lack of certain customary standards. Uncertainties about a possible cause and effect should be expressed to the patient's family. Explicit acknowledgment of an error, its consequences, and therapeutic measures to reduce further harm should be discussed in a separate meeting with the family. Adequate documentation, disclosure, and candor should be part of standard care.

Putting It All Together

- Physicians are biased in favor of simple diagnoses and simple solutions.
- Recognition of possible errors requires communication of the ED with the neurology department.
- Major diagnostic errors can be taught for avoidance.
- The top three diagnostic errors are failure to appreciate mass effect and hydrocephalus, basilar artery embolus, and ischemic stroke with vertigo.
- Error management is equally important and improves performance.

References

1. Agarwal R, Manandhar L, Saluja P, Grandhi B. Pontine stroke presenting as isolated facial nerve palsy mimicking Bell's palsy: a case report. *J Med Case Rep* 2011;5:287.
2. Berner ES, Graber ML. Overconfidence as a cause of diagnostic error in medicine. *Am J Med* 2008;121:S2–23.
3. Bo SH, Davidsen EM, Gulbrandsen P, Dietrichs E. Acute headache: a prospective diagnostic work-up of patients admitted to a general hospital. *Eur J Neurol* 2008;15:1293–1299.
4. Chowdhury FA, Nashef L, Elwes RD. Misdiagnosis in epilepsy: a review and recognition of diagnostic uncertainty. *Eur J Neurol* 2008;15:1034–1042.
5. Croskerry P. Cognitive and affective dispositions to respond. In: Croskerry P, Cosby K, Schenkel S, Wears R, eds. *Patient Safety in Emergency Medicine*. Philadelphia, PA: Lippincott Williams & Wilkins; 2009:219–227.
6. Croskerry PG. Avoiding pitfalls in the emergency room. *Canadian Journal of CME* 1996:63–76.
7. Dugas AF, Lucas JM, Edlow JA. Diagnosis of spinal cord compression in nontrauma patients in the emergency department. *Acad Emerg Med* 2011;18:719–725.
8. Edlow JA, Malek AM, Ogilvy CS. Aneurysmal subarachnoid hemorrhage: update for emergency physicians. *J Emerg Med* 2008;34:237–251.
9. Edlow JA. Diagnosis of subarachnoid hemorrhage. *Neurocrit Care* 2005;2:99–109.
10. Elstein AS. Clinical reasoning in medicine. In: Higgs J, Jones M, eds. *Clinical Reasoning in the Health Professions*. Oxford, England: Butterworth-Heinemann; 1995:49–59.
11. Ely JW, Graber ML, Croskerry P. Checklists to reduce diagnostic errors. *Acad Med* 2011;86:307–313.
12. Fahimi J, Navi BB, Kamel H. Potential misdiagnoses of Bell's palsy in the emergency department. *Ann Emerg Med* 2014;63:428–434.
13. Gifford DR, Mittman BS, Vickrey BG. Diagnostic reasoning in neurology. *Neurol Clin* 1996;14:223–238.
14. Groopman J. *How Doctors Think*. Houghton Mifflin; 2007.
15. Hansen CK, Fisher J, Joyce N, Edlow JA. Emergency department consultations for patients with neurological emergencies. *Eur J Neurol* 2011;18:1317–1322.

16. Helmreich RL. On error management: lessons from aviation. *BMJ* 2000;320:781–785.
17. Jalloh I, Minhas P. Delays in the treatment of cauda equina syndrome due to its variable clinical features in patients presenting to the emergency department. *Emerg Med J* 2007;24:33–34.
18. Kahneman D, Tversky A. On the psychology of prediction. *Psychological Review* 1973;80:237–251.
19. Kim AS, Fullerton HJ, Johnston SC. Risk of vascular events in emergency department patients discharged home with diagnosis of dizziness or vertigo. *Ann Emerg Med* 2011;57:34–41.
20. Laurent A, Aubert L, Chahraoui K, et al. Error in intensive care: psychological repercussions and defense mechanisms among health professionals. *Crit Care Med* 2014;42:2370–2378.
21. Lee H, Sohn SI, Cho YW, et al. Cerebellar infarction presenting isolated vertigo: frequency and vascular topographical patterns. *Neurology* 2006;67:1178–1183.
22. Moeller JJ, Kurniawan J, Gubitz GJ, Ross JA, Bhan V. Diagnostic accuracy of neurological problems in the emergency department. *Can J Neurol Sci* 2008;35:335–341.
23. Moulin T, Sablot D, Vidry E, et al. Impact of emergency room neurologists on patient management and outcome. *Eur Neurol* 2003;50:207–214.
24. Redelmeier DA. Improving patient care: the cognitive psychology of missed diagnoses. *Ann Intern Med* 2005;142:115–120.
25. Rothschild JM, Churchill W, Erickson A, et al. Medication errors recovered by emergency department pharmacists. *Ann Emerg Med* 2010;55:513–521.
26. Royl G, Ploner CJ, Leithner C. Dizziness in the emergency room: diagnoses and misdiagnoses. *Eur Neurol* 2011;66:256–263.
27. Schrock JW, Glasenapp M, Victor A, Losey T, Cydulka RK. Variables associated with discordance between emergency physician and neurologist diagnoses of transient ischemic attacks in the emergency department. *Ann Emerg Med* 2012;59:19–26.
28. Seibert HH, Maddox RR, Flynn EA, Williams CK. Effect of barcode technology with electronic medication administration record on medication accuracy rates. *Am J Health Syst Pharm* 2014;71:209–218.
29. Sloman SA. The empirical case for two systems of reasoning. *Psychological Bulletin* 1996;119:3–22.
30. Stangierski A, Warmuz-Stangierska I, Ruchala M, et al. Medical errors—not only patients' problem. *Arch Med Sci* 2012;8:569–574.
31. Stasiak P, Afilalo M, Castelino T, et al. Detection and correction of prescription errors by an emergency department pharmacy service. *CJEM* 2014;16:193–206.
32. Tversky A, Kahneman D. Rational choice and the framing of decisions. *J Business* 1986;59:S251.
33. Vermeulen MJ, Schull MJ. Missed diagnosis of subarachnoid hemorrhage in the emergency department. *Stroke* 2007;38:1216–1221.
34. Vickrey BG, Samuels MA, Ropper AH. How neurologists think: a cognitive psychology perspective on missed diagnoses. *Ann Neurol* 2010;67:425–433.
35. Wears RL, Wu AW. Dealing with failure: the aftermath of errors and adverse events. *Ann Emerg Med* 2002;39:344–346.
36. West CP, Huschka MM, Novotny PJ, et al. Association of perceived medical errors with resident distress and empathy: a prospective longitudinal study. *JAMA* 2006;296:1071–1078.
37. Wu AW, Folkman S, McPhee SJ, et al. Do house officers learn from their mistakes? *JAMA* 265:2089–2094, 1991.
38. Wu AW. Medical error: the second victim. The doctor who makes the mistake needs help too. *BMJ* 2000;320:726–727.

Index